Nadinia Davis, MBA, CIA, CPA, RHIA

Assistant Professor
Health Information Management
Kean University
Union, New Jersey

Melissa LaCour, RHIA

Program Director
Health Information Technology
Delgado Community College
New Orleans, Louisiana

*Study Guide to Accompany*

# Introduction to

# Health Information Technology

**W.B. SAUNDERS COMPANY**

*A Harcourt Health Sciences Company*

Philadelphia · London · New York · St. Louis · Sydney · Toronto

W.B. SAUNDERS COMPANY
*A Harcourt Health Sciences Company*
The Curtis Center
Independence Square West
Philadelphia, Pennsylvania 19106-3399

*Study Guide to Accompany*
*Introduction to Health Information Technology*          ISBN 0-7216-8354-1

Printed in the United States of America

Last digit is the print number: 9 8 7 6 5 4 3 2 1

362.1068
D2611

# Table of Contents

# How to Use This Study Guide

The purpose of this study guide is to help you remember, understand, and apply the information in the accompanying text: *Introduction to Health Information Technology*. The study guide is divided into chapters that correspond to the text. Each study guide chapter is divided into sections. Learners can use those sections to study, as follows:

## Up to Speed Notes

This section is a review of elements that were covered in the text chapter. It provides memory joggers that will help you to recall the text material. After you have read the text, use this section to ensure that you have absorbed the text material. Read each bullet, recalling the information in the text. Each bullet ends with a prompt for you to finish a list or a description, or to give examples of the items discussed. If you can't recall the information, refer back to the text to refresh your memory.

## Vocabulary/Review Questions

This section contains fill-ins, multiple choice, matching, and short-answer questions. After you have read the text and reviewed with the Up to Speed Notes, use this section to test your knowledge of the text material. The answers to the questions in this section are in the back of this Study Guide.

## Critical Thinking Exercises

These questions and activities are designed to help you apply the text material to practical questions. Some of the questions will require you to think about what you learned in previous text Chapters and connect it to the current Chapter material.

## What Else Is Available?

The companion web site contains documents and links to sites that support the text Chapter material and Critical Thinking exercises. Documents and links that pertain specifically to the current chapter are referenced here. By reading the chapter, reviewing the chapter material, and self-testing, you can master the text chapter material efficiently. If you are using the text in conjunction with a course, your instructor may supplement the text material with additional information. Use of this study guide can help you build a good foundation on which to add that additional material.

# 1

# Health Care Delivery Systems

## Up to Speed Notes

- Physicians must complete extensive courses of study in medicine and their individual specialties. There are numerous physician specialties. Specialties may correspond to the activities that the physician performs, such as surgery or radiology. Other specialties focus on the study of a particular body system, such as urology, or a specific disease, such as oncology. List as many medical specialties as you can remember and describe what they do. Refer to Table 1-1 in the text to see how well you did.
- Physicians diagnose diseases and perform certain procedures, both diagnostic and therapeutic. Distinguish between diagnosis and procedure. Give examples of both.
- Much of the care for patients is performed by various Allied Health Professionals. List as many allied health professionals as you can remember and describe what they do. Refer to Table 1-3 in the text to see how well you did.
- The fundamental difference between ambulatory care and acute care is the patient's length of stay. Ambulatory patients are called 'outpatients' and acute care patients are called 'inpatients'. In your own words, describe the differences between the two. What problems arise in an acute care facility in distinguishing between an outpatient and an inpatient? What are some other differences between ambulatory care and acute care?
- Health care facilities can be compared in many ways other than length of stay: Organizational structure and ownership are two of those ways. List and describe in your own words how facilities can be different from each other.
- We mentioned several types of health care settings. List as many different settings as you can remember. Identify and distinguish between health care settings.
- The time that an inpatient stays in the hospital is referred to as Length of Stay. How do we calculate Length of Stay? Average Length of Stay?
- Health care facilities must be licensed in order to conduct business. However, they often choose to be accredited as well. What is licensure? What is accreditation? What is the difference between licensure and accreditation?
- There are many different organizations that accredit health care facilities and educational programs. List as many accrediting bodies that you can remember and which facilities or programs they accredit.
- Government is involved in health care as both a regulator and a payer. Describe how government regulates and pays for health care. What levels of government are involved in these activities?

# Vocabulary

1. "Diabetes" is an example of a _____.

2. A health care organization that has permanent facilities, 24-hour nursing care, and an organized medical staff is a type of _____.

3. A hospital with an average length of stay less than 30 days, an emergency department, operating suite, and clinical departments to handle a broad range of diagnoses and treatments is most likely an _____.

4. A specialty inpatient facility that focuses on the treatment of individuals who are not adults is a _____.

5. An _____ provides care to patients at all or most points along the continuum of care.

6. Care for the terminally ill is the focus of _____ care.

7. Health care professionals must adhere to their discipline's _____.

8. _____ focuses on treating patients where they reside.

9. Medicare waives compliance audits for appropriately accredited facilities by granting them _____.

10. Occupational therapy is an example of an _____.

11. Patients whose care requires them to remain in the hospital overnight are called _____.

12. The actual number of beds that a hospital has available for inpatients is called the _____.

13. The broad range of services that may be required by a patient in his/her lifetime is referred to as the _____.

14. Voluntary compliance with a set of standards developed by an independent agency is part of the _____ process.

15. When one physician asks another physician for an opinion regarding the care of a patient, the first physician is asking for a _____.

## Multiple Choice

1. A patient was admitted to the hospital on September 13 and discharged on September 30. What is the length of stay?
   A. 13 days
   B. 17 days
   C. 18 days
   D. 30 days

2. A patient was admitted to the hospital on August 20 and discharged on October 6. What is the length of stay?
   A. 47 days
   B. 48 days
   C. 66 days
   D. 67 days

3. The Community Care Center has 200 beds. It has an average length of stay of 2 years. Most of the patients are elderly, but there are some younger patients with serious chronic illnesses. Community Care Center is most likely a(n):
   A. Acute Care facility
   B. Behavioral health facility
   C. Long-term care facility
   D. Rehabilitation facility

4. Another term for a Consultation is a(n):
   A. Therapy
   B. Referral
   C. Operation
   D. Encounter

5. Chapone Health Care is an organization that owns a number of different health care facilities: three acute care hospitals, two long-term care facilities, and a number of physician offices. Chapone also owns a rehabilitation hospital and an assisted living facility, which also delivers home care. They deliver care to patients at every point along the continuum of care. Chapone Health Care can be described as a(n):
   A. Hospital
   B. Chain
   C. Fiscal Intermediary
   D. Integrated Health Care Delivery System

6. The following patients were discharged from pediatrics for the week 7/16/01–7/22/01:

| Patient Name | Admission Date | Discharge Date |
|---|---|---|
| Groot | 7/13/01 | 7/15/01 |
| Smith | 7/12/01 | 7/15/01 |
| Brown | 7/11/01 | 7/16/01 |
| Kowalski | 7/10/01 | 7/20/01 |
| Zhong | 7/09/01 | 7/19/01 |
| Frank | 6/29/01 | 7/18/01 |

The average length of stay of these patients is:

A. 6.5 days
B. 7 days
C. 7.2 days
D. 8 days

7. Which of the following is NOT an agency within the Department of Health and Human Services?

A. FDA
B. HCFA
C. NIH
D. OSHA

8. Medicare is administered by:

A. FDA
B. HCFA
C. Individual States
D. NCQA

9. A facility that focuses totally on palliative care is a(n):

A. Ambulatory care facility
B. Hospice
C. Long-term care facility
D. Managed care

10. Which of the following is an example of a diagnosis?

A. Tonsillitis
B. Appendectomy
C. Chest x-ray
D. Physical therapy

11. Which of the following is an example of a procedure?

A. Diabetes
B. Pneumonia
C. Tonsillectomy
D. Appendicitis

12. Which of the following qualifies an acute care facility for 'deemed status'?

A. State licensure
B. CARF accreditation
C. JCAHO accreditation
D. Compliance with COP

# Matching

Match the diagnosis, activity, or patient group on the left with the name of the specialty on the right.

| | |
|---|---|
| 1. Administers substances that cause loss of sensation. | A. Allergist |
| 2. Cancer patients. | B. Anesthesiologist |
| 3. Care related to the female reproductive system. | C. Cardiologist |
| 4. Cares for women before, during, and after delivery. | D. Dermatologist |
| 5. Delivers primary health care for children. | E. Family practitioner |
| 6. Delivers primary health care for patients of all ages. | F. Gastroenterologist |
| 7. Diseases and abnormal conditions of newborns. | G. Gynecologist |
| 8. Diseases of the digestive system. | H. Neonatologist |
| 9. Diseases of the heart and blood vessels. | I. Obstetrician |
| 10. Diseases of the muscles and bones. | J. Oncologist |
| 11. Diseases of the skin. | K. Ophthalmologist |
| 12. Disorders of the mind. | L. Orthopedist |
| 13. Eye diseases. | M. Pathologist |
| 14. Patients who have strong reactions to pollen and insect bites. | N. Pediatrician |
| 15. Studies changes in cells, tissue, and organs. | O. Psychiatrist |

Match accrediting bodies on the left with the type of organization on the right. Some accrediting bodies accredit more than one type of organization.

| | |
|---|---|
| 1. AAAHC | A. Acute Care |
| 2. AOA | B. Ambulatory Care Facilities |
| 3. CARF | C. Home Health Care |
| 4. CHAP | D. Managed Care Organizations |
| 5. JCAHO | E. Osteopathic Hospitals |
| 6. NCQA | F. Rehabilitation Facilities |

## Critical Thinking Exercises

1. If you were just diagnosed with diabetes, how would you go about finding a physician to care for you?

2. Identify a facility in your area by looking in the telephone book or on the Internet. Find out as much as you can about the facility, including the types of services it offers. Describe the facility in terms of size, organization, patients, and average length of stay. What type of facility is it?

3. Log on to the AHIMA website (www.ahima.org). Explore the site. What does AHIMA say about careers in Health Information Management? How many schools offer degrees in Health Information Management? What courses are included in these programs?

4. What is the difference between Occupational Therapy and Physical Therapy? If you have trouble explaining the difference, try logging on to the Internet and find the websites for their national professional associations. What do those sites have to offer the public in terms of information about the profession?

## What Else Is Available?

The companion site has links to various government agencies, health care facilities, and professional associations. Check these out to find out more information about the health care industry.

# 2

# Data Elements

## Up to Speed Notes

▶ Health is not merely the absence of disease. In your own words, describe what conditions must exist in order for a person to be 'healthy'.

▶ The fundamental difference between data and information is that information is presented in a frame of reference. Give two examples of how data becomes information.

▶ Health data and health information relate to the health care industry. We may be considering the data about a single individual or many individuals. Give two examples of how health data becomes health information.

▶ The ambulatory care environment is easiest for us to understand, because it is the environment to which we are most frequently exposed. Physicians, nurses, medical secretaries, and a variety of health information management professionals provide services to ambulatory care patients. Describe the experiences of a patient in a physician's office. What professionals is the patient likely to encounter? What role do those professionals play in caring for the patient?

▶ There are four general categories of health data: demographic, socioeconomic, financial, and clinical. We collect this data in order to identify the patient, understand the patient's history and present circumstances, confirm who will pay for the care that is rendered to the patient, and investigate the patient's health status. Describe what data is collected in each category and list two examples of each type of data.

▶ In ambulatory care, data begins to be collected when the patient makes an appointment. More data is collected at the time of patient registration and throughout the visit. Describe the collection of data in the ambulatory care environment. What is collected and by whom?

▶ The Uniform Ambulatory Care Data Set is a list of data elements that Medicare requires to be collected about all patients treated in this environment for whom Medicare reimbursement is sought. List and describe the elements of the UACDS.

▶ In collecting data, we must identify it and compile it in such a way that it can be communicated between health care providers and other individuals and organizations. In order to properly define and describe this data, we collect it in fully defined fields, which are further combined into records. Define characters, fields, records, and files. Give two examples of each.

# Vocabulary

1. A single letter, number, or symbol is a _____.

2. The study of disease trends and occurrences is _____.

3. The quality that data reflects the known or acceptable range of values for the specific data is called _____.

4. The quality of data being correct is called _____.

5. A collection or series of related characters is a _____.

6. Data collected for the purpose of patient identification is _____.

7. Data collected during the investigation of the patient's current health situation is called _____.

8. In a database, a list of details about each field is a _____.

9. The smallest element or unit of knowledge is _____.

10. After all other payment sources are exhausted, the _____ is responsible for the remaining balance of payments.

11. The initial collection of height, weight, temperature, and blood pressure on a patient's first visit to a physician is called _____ data.

12. Data which pertain to the patient's personal life and personal habits, such as marital status and religion, are _____.

13. Data collected about the party who will pay for the patient's health care is _____.

## Multiple Choice

1. Which of the following is a symptom?
   A. Diabetes mellitus
   B. Lung cancer
   C. Runny nose
   D. Asthma

2. The ability of a patient to see a physician without an appointment is called:
   A. Appointment-free
   B. Open-access
   C. Free scheduling
   D. Open appointments

3. Which of the following is an example of demographic data?
   A. Address
   B. Marital status
   C. Race
   D. Employer

4. Another term for a Demographic data is:
   A. Explanatory
   B. Referral
   C. Global
   D. Indicative

5. Of the following workers in a physician's office, who is the most likely one to collect the patient's blood pressure?
   A. Physician
   B. Nurse
   C. Medical secretary
   D. Health information technician

6. Which of the following is NOT an example of clinical data?
   A. Appendectomy three years ago
   B. Smokes 2 packs of cigarettes daily
   C. Blood pressure
   D. Wears glasses to read

7. If a patient's insurance company has reimbursed the physician for the appropriate amount and there is still a balance due in the patient's account, the physician must apply next for payment to the:
   A. Guarantor
   B. State government
   C. Medicaid
   D. Patient's parents

8. Which of the following is an example of a field?

A. J

B. NJ

C. New Jersey

D. All of the above

USE THE SAMPLE DATA DICTIONARY BELOW TO ANSWER QUESTIONS 9 - 10

| Name | Definition | Size | Type | Example |
|------|------------|------|------|---------|
| FNAME | Patient's First Name | 15 Characters | Alphabetic | Jane |
| LNAME | Patient's Last Name | 15 Characters | Alphabetic | Jones |
| HTEL | Patient's Home Telephone Number | 12 Characters | Alpha-numeric | 973-555-3331 |
| TEMP | Patient's Temperature | 5 Characters | Numeric | 98.6 |

9. Using 12 alpha-numeric characters is one way to capture the patient's home telephone number. List at least one other way to capture that data.

10. List and describe two additional fields that would be needed to capture a patient's entire name.

11. Using the format above, define the fields that would be needed to capture a patient's diagnosis and a procedure. Refer to Chapter One for examples that you can use.

## Matching

Match the physician office activity described on the left with the name of the professional most likely to perform it on the right.

1. Administers allergy shots
2. Answers telephone and records appointments
3. Draws blood for diagnostic testing
4. Handles billing and requests for patient information
5. Queries patient as to reason for encounter, takes vital signs

A.   Health information technician

B.   Medical assistant

C.   Medical secretary

D.   Phlebotomist

E.   Registered nurse

## Critical Thinking Exercises

1. How does the quantity of health data impact our understanding of what it contains?

2. How can a large quantity of health data be communicated in a meaningful way (as information)?

3. The Uniform Ambulatory Care Data Set (UACDS) is a list of data elements that Medicare requires to be collected about all patients treated in this environment for whom Medicare reimbursement is sought. List and describe the elements of the UACDS. Who collects this data and when is it collected?

4. In order to properly define and describe health data, we collect it in fully defined fields, which are further combined into records. The UACDS is an example of a list of fields. When compiled about a single patient, that patient's data becomes a record in the UACDS file. For each data element in the UACDS, define the field that describes that data element. Arrange your responses in simple, data dictionary format.

## What Else Is Available?

The companion site contains links to various web sites that will help you obtain further information about the discussions in this chapter.

# 3
# Organization of Data Elements in a Health Record

## Up to Speed Notes

▶ The data collection devices (forms) in paper-based records are organized into folders in one of three ways: by date, by source or preparer, or by patient problem/diagnosis. What are the technical names for these methods? In which health care facilities are these methods most likely to be used?

▶ Physicians collect and record their notes in a structure that helps the reader to identify the patient's perceptions, the physician's observations, the physician's diagnostic impression and treatment plan. What is the acronym for this structure? What do the letters in the acronym mean? Give an example of what might be in a physician's note under each letter.

▶ Upon admission, patient data is collected which helps to identify the patient and the payer for the services to be rendered. List as many data items (fields) as you can recall that would be included in an admission record.

▶ From admission to discharge, the patient moves through a health care facility in a predictable pattern of events. Tests and therapies are conducted by a variety of personnel, and many different services are rendered to the patient. Describe the events that will occur when a patient is admitted to an acute care facility for an operation. What caregivers will be involved with the patient?

▶ A data collection device, in the context of this Chapter, is a paper-based form or computer-based screen on which individuals record specific data about a patient. Data collection devices help health care workers record valid data accurately. How can data collection devices affect the quality of data? Give examples.

▶ In this Chapter, we discussed some of the actual data collection devices that are used in health care facilities, particularly acute care. Table 3-7 lists the key items in a physician order. List those items as fields and describe them in data dictionary format, as discussed in Chapter 2.

▶ There are some differences in the considerations in developing paper-based versus computer-based data capture devices. List as many differences as you remember.

▶ Medicare requires a specific list of data elements to be collected about each patient who is discharged from an acute care facility. This list is called the Uniform Hospital Discharge Data Set (UHDDS). List as many items as you can remember from the UHDDS.

## Vocabulary

1.  A physician who only performs operations is a _____.

2.  Another was to refer to a form is as a _____.

3.  Another word for therapy is _____.

4.  At the end of a hospital stay, a _____ is usually required to be completed, often as a dictated and transcribed report.

5.  If a health care professional is working under the supervision of another, such as a resident being supervised by an attending physician, then the notes written by that professional must be _____ by the supervisor.

6.  In medical decision making, the physician's evaluation of the subjective and objective evidence is called the _____

7.  In order to _____ a document other data collection device, a physician may sign the document or enter a password.

8.  Routine documentation of the nurse's interaction with a patient is recorded in the _____.

9.  Sometimes a physician needs to ask another physician for an opinion regarding the care of a patient. The physician whom he asks is referred to as the _____.

10. The act of rendering an opinion about another physician's patient is called a _____.

11. The cause or source of a patient's condition or disease is called the _____.

12. The first page in a paper record is usually the _____.

13. The physician who is primarily responsible for coordinating the care of the patient in the hospital is the _____.

14. When a patient is first seen by a physician in any health care setting, the physician generally records the patient's chief complaint, pertinent family and social data, and a review of the patient's body systems. This record is called the _____.

15. When paper records are organized in chronological order, they are described as: _____.

## Multiple Choice

1. Which of the following is an element of an acute care admission record?
   A. Patient's previous operations
   B. Type of dwelling in which the patient lives
   C. Name of patient's employer
   D. Patient's height and weight

2. Which of the following data elements is NOT likely to appear on an acute care admission record?
   A. Patient's religion
   B. Patient's date of birth
   C. Name of the patient's spouse
   D. Tobacco use by the patient

3. If a hospital wanted to correspond with a patient after discharge, the appropriate source of the patient's current address would be the:
   A. Discharge summary
   B. Attending physician's office records
   C. History & Physical
   D. Latest admission record

4. Which of the following is not a necessary part of a medication record?
   A. Physician's signature
   B. Description of the physician's order
   C. Nurses' signatures
   D. Data and time of administration of drug

5. Which of the following is an example of the 'P' in SOAP?
   A. Pancreatitis versus hiatal hernia versus gastritis
   B. Patient reports continued pain in the abdomen, particularly after eating.
   C. Patient's abdomen is tender to palpation in the epigastric region.
   D. Schedule barium swallow.

6. Which of the following is an example of the 'O' in SOAP?
   A. Pancreatitis versus hiatal hernia versus gastritis
   B. Patient reports continued pain in the abdomen, particularly after eating.
   C. Patient's abdomen is tender to palpation in the epigastric region.
   D. Schedule barium swallow.

7. The nursing department in your facility has submitted a form to the forms committee for approval. The form is printed on dark gold paper so that it will stand out in the chart. You recommend a light yellow paper instead, because it photocopies better than dark gold. This is an example of taking into consideration:
   A. The purpose of the data collection device
   B. The needs of all users of the device
   C. An understanding of the technology used
   D. Simplicity

8. The purpose of instructions on a data collection device is to:
   A. Ensure that the correct form is used
   B. Help users with complicated data collection
   C. Help ensure the consistency of data collection
   D. Sequence the data collection correctly

9. All of the following are elements of the UHDDS EXCEPT:
   A. Principal diagnosis
   B. Race
   C. Marital Status
   D. Disposition

10. When entering physician orders in a computer-based system, the computer can check the authentication to ensure that the individual who entered the data is authorized to do so (that is, that the authentication is correct). This is an example of a computer being used to ensure data:
    A. Validity
    B. Accuracy
    C. Completeness
    D. Timeliness

## Matching

Match the physician progress note entry on the left with the SOAP note component on the right.

1. 60 mg. Pseudoephedrine, every 4 hours. 100 mg. Tylenol, as needed for pain.
2. Acute sinusitis with pharyngitis.
3. Patient complaints of headache.
4. Patient's frontal sinuses are sensitive to percussion. Lungs are clear. Throat is slightly inflamed.

A. Subjective
B. Objective
C. Assessment
D. Plan

Match the chart description on the left with the record order on the right.

1. All of the information about the patient's Congestive Heart Failure is together, the Hypertension information is all together, and the Appendicitis information is all together.
2. Data is collected and recorded by different health care workers and linked to other data about the patient by common data elements.
3. In the record, all of the physician's notes are together, the orders are together, the nursing notes are together, the medication sheets are together, and the laboratory reports are together.
4. The record is organized in chronological order only.

A. Integrated
B. Source-oriented
C. Problem-oriented
D. Computer-based

Match the definition on the left with the Vocabulary word(s) on the right.

1. Acronym that describes the medical decision-making process. Also refers to the way physicians organize their progress notes.
2. Analysis of body fluids.
3. Examination of a patient using x-rays.
4. One or more surgical procedures performed at the same time.
5. Record of all drugs given to a patient during the hospitalization.
6. The diagnostic, therapeutic, or palliative measures that will be taken to investigate or treat the patient's condition or disease.
7. The nurse's evaluation of the patient.
8. The physician's directions regarding the patient's care. Also refers to the data collection device on which these elements are captured.
9. The physician's documentation of a surgical procedure, usually dictated and transcribed.
10. The physician's documentation of the examination of the patient, particularly at the initial visit.
11. The physician's record of each visit with the patient.
12. The predetermined, routine orders that have been designated to pertain to specific diagnoses or procedures. Must be ordered and authenticated by the appropriate physician.
13. The process of systematically eliminating potential diagnoses. Also refers to the list of potential diagnoses.

A. Laboratory tests
B. Medication sheet
C. Nursing assessment
D. Operation
E. Operative report
F. Physical exam
G. Physician's orders
H. Plan of treatment
I. Progress notes
J. Radiology tests
K. Rule out
L. SOAP format
M. Standing orders

## Critical Thinking Exercises

1. Identify an acute care facility in your area by looking in the telephone book or on the internet. Find out as much as you can about the facility, including the types of services it offers. Describe the facility in terms of size, organization, patients, and average length of stay.

2. Compare and contrast the physician's SOAP strategy of documentation with the nursing strategy of documentation. Why are they different?

3. In an acute care facility, only the physician's documentation is considered when applying for Medicare reimbursement. Why isn't nursing documentation considered?

4. In a long-term care facility, the physician's documentation is considered, but the nursing and therapy documentation are also very important when applying for Medicare reimbursement. Why do you think reimbursement for acute care is different than reimbursement for long-term care?

5. Figure 3-10 is an example of a paper-based physician order form. Using what you know about the data elements in this form, how would you create a computer screen to capture the order? Could you use the data entry process to improve the accuracy, validity, and completeness of the data as it is entered? How?

6. Based on your answers to Question 5, who do you think should be allowed to enter the physician order into the computer? Describe both the authors and the authentication procedures that you would require.

7. List the elements of the Uniform Hospital Discharge Data Set (UHDDS) in data dictionary format, as described in Chapter Two. For each item, list the source of the data element (the individual in the facility who first collects the data element).

8. Compare and contrast the UACDS with the UHDDS. Why are they different?

9. Based on what you learned about Long-Term Care (LTC) facilities in Chapter One, how would you expect data collection to be different there, compared to acute care facilities? Considering the length of stay and the type of care delivered, what would you expect to be included in the LTC data set, compared to the UHDDS?

## What Else Is Available?

The companion site has examples of both paper-based and computer-based data collection devices. Try answering Questions 5 and 6 using other data collection devices.

# 4

# Postdischarge
# Processing

## Up to Speed Notes

- Maintaining high standards of data quality is essential for patient care and effective other uses of health data. Data quality has a number of characteristics, many of which were discussed in this Chapter and the preceding Chapters. List and define as many characteristics as you can remember.
- Protection of data quality and integrity is aided by the development and implementation of internal controls. We discussed three fundamental types of internal controls. List and define them.
- Health Information Management professionals perform a variety of internal control tasks within the context of postdischarge processing. List and describe one example of each type of control that is performed during this process.
- In a paper environment, records must physically move from the patient care area to the HIM Department for processing and storage. Give two examples of how that movement can occur.
- When the HIM Department obtains control of the records, a process must be in place to determine whether all records have been received.
- There is a logical order to postdischarge processing. List the postdischarge processing steps, in order, beginning with obtaining control of the record.
- Analyzing a record is the first step in the incomplete record system. Name the subsequent steps and the purpose of each step.

## Vocabulary

1. A computer can create a log of processing and access activities called an _____.

2. A detective control function designed to identify incomplete data in a record is _____.

3. A list of deficient or other problem data, usually generated by a computer, is an _____.

4. A list of potentially inaccurate or problem data, usually generated by a computer, is an _____.

5. A paper record must be _____ before it can be analyzed.

6. Another word for an Incomplete System is a _____.

7. Assignment of ICD-9-CM codes to clinical data while the patient is still being treated is _____.

8. Clinicians can evidence supervision of subordinate personnel by _____ the subordinates documentation.

9. Data that has been obtained, recorded, and/or reported within a predetermined period satisfies the data quality characteristic of _____.

10. In a paper record environment, _____ refers to the maintenance of the same page order both pre- and postdischarge.

11. Parts of paper records that arrive in the HIM Department separately from the main record are often called _____.

12. Required elements of a record that are missing are called _____.

13. _____ procedures govern the storage of records, including duration, location, security, and access.

14. The data quality characteristic of data being present or existing in its entirety is _____.

15. The process of recording elements into a collection device is called _____.

16. The purpose of _____ is to review the chart while the patient is still being treated.

## Multiple Choice

1. Which of the following is a detective control?
   A. Alerting a physician that a patient is allergic to an ordered medication.
   B. Reviewing a chart to ensure that medications were administered on a timely basis.
   C. The HIM Department sends a physician a list of her incomplete charts.
   D. A coder reviews a record in order to assign a clinical code.

2. The coding system used to track diagnoses and procedures in an acute care setting is:
   A. ICD-9-CM
   B. ICD-O
   C. DSM-IV
   D. CPT-4

3. Which of the following is an example of a nomenclature?
   A. ICD-9-CM
   B. ICD-O
   C. CPT-4
   D. DRG

4. All of the following are steps in postdischarge processing EXCEPT:
   A. Coding
   B. Abstracting
   C. Chart retrieval
   D. Concurrent analysis

5. Which of the following is a preventive control?
   A. Alerting a physician that a patient is allergic to an ordered medication.
   B. Reviewing a chart to ensure that medications were administered on a timely basis.
   C. The HIM Department sends a physician a list of her incomplete charts.
   D. A coder reviews a record in order to assign a clinical code.

6. Upon review of a record, the analyst determines that the physician has not signed several progress notes. This record fails to reflect the data quality characteristic of:
   A. Accuracy
   B. Timeliness
   C. Completeness
   D. B&C

7. The JCAHO requires that acute care records be completed:
   A. Within 15 days of discharge
   B. In whatever time period the facility requires
   C. Within 30 days of discharge
   D. In whatever time period the State requires

8. Acute care facilities are permitted to have delinquent records, but the number of delinquent records must not exceed:
   A. 2% of average monthly discharges
   B. 50 records
   C. 50% of average monthly discharges
   D. 9 records

9. Which of the following is a corrective control?
   A. A nurse alerts the physician that the patient is allergic to an ordered medication.
   B. The nursing supervisor reviews a record to ensure that medications were administered correctly.
   C. The HIM Department sends a physician a list of her incomplete charts.
   D. A coder reviews a record in order to assign a clinical code.

10. Community Hospital, an acute care facility, is preparing for a Joint Commission survey. The Chief Operating Officer is reviewing the following data from the Health Information Management Department:

| Month | # Discharges | # Delinquent Records |
|---|---|---|
| January | 1000 | 450 |
| February | 1200 | 600 |
| March | 1100 | 500 |
| April | 1100 | 600 |

What is Community Hospital's average monthly discharges?

   A. 538
   B. 1000
   C. 1100
   D. 1200

11. How many delinquent records is Community Hospital permitted to have?
   A. 450
   B. 500
   C. 550
   D. 600

12. At the end of April, is Community Hospital in compliance with JCAHO rules?
   A. Yes
   B. No
   C. Not enough information is given to answer the question.

13. Control over records in process can be maintained using:
   A. Batch control record and deficiency sheets
   B. Central staging area and deficiency sheets
   C. Batch control record and central staging area
   D. Deficiency sheets and loose sheets

## Critical Thinking Exercises

1. You have just checked in all of the records received from the nursing unit. One record that was received is not on your discharge register. What could have happened? How would you determine what to do with the extra record?

2. Based on your knowledge of rehabilitation and long-term care, how do you think documentation issues and HIM processing issues differ in these facilities from those in acute care?

3. What internal control roles are played in the Health Information Management department? Your answer should include, but not be limited to, identification of the function and the specific internal control role that it plays.

4. What is the purpose of a discharge register? How is it used in postdischarge processing? How else could it be used?

5. Since the HIM department is primarily concerned with postdischarge processing, of what use is the Admission Register to this department?

6. List the forms that are present, in one form or another, in every acute care health record. How would you organize those forms in a record while it is in the nursing unit? Postdischarge? Why do you think some organizations want the record to be organized differently pre- and postdischarge?

7. What processing problems can occur if an organization implements a universal chart order? How is the issue of record organization resolved in a computer-based record?

8. Is a computer-based record completely paperless? Why or why not?

## What Else Is Available?

The companion site has sample forms and computer screens. You can print some of these out and practice assembling a paper record or make a 'sample record' for study purposes.

# 5

# Storage of Health Data

## Up to Speed Notes

▶ Health information, whether paper or computer based, must be stored in an organized, secure environment for the duration of the retention schedule.

▶ The Master Patient Index, MPI, is a tool in the health care facility used to store unique identifiable information on each patient who has been registered in that facility. The MPI is especially useful in a facility that uses a numerical system to identify patient records, because the MPI correlates the patient to the MR#. List the desired content of a computerized MPI. Table 5-1 reviews the suggested content of a computerized MPI.

▶ The physical file folder that contains the health care records must be labeled for identification. The identification can either be alphabetic or numeric. List and describe each of the numeric identification systems. Review Table 5-4 for the pros and cons of each.

▶ In the paper based health care record, a numerical identification system used to identify the file is also used to organize the files within a filing system. List and describe the different filing methods. Review Table 5-7.

▶ Computer based records are identified using an index for organized retrieval within the computer system.

▶ Because space is often limited in the facility, health care records may be maintained in alternative storage methods. List and explain each of the methods discussed in Chapter 5.

▶ Health care records are stored in various file furniture. List and describe the filing furniture used to store paper-based health care records. What measurements are important in the design of a file area? Review Table 5-9.

▶ Health care records must be maintained for a specific number of years. Do you recall how to determine the number of years a group of health care records must be maintained?

▶ Explain what measures can be taken to protect health care records from: Fire, water damage, theft, and tampering.

▶ It is important for the Health Information Management Department to locate records in timely manner. Can you identify and describe the system used to locate medical records within a facility?

# Vocabulary

1. A digital form of the patient's paper health care record is called the _____.

2. _____ is an alternative storage method for paper records using computer-based methods.

3. An _____ is used to identify or name a file or record so that it can be located in the computer based health record.

4. The numerical file identification system used to identify an entire family's health record using one number and modifiers is called _____.

5. The length of time that a record must be retained is called the _____.

6. _____ and _____ are alternative storage methods for paper records using plastic film.

7. A _____ is used to identify the location of records within a facility.

8. The physical container used to store the paper based health record is a _____.

9. A _____ is a compilation of patient health information, and various media forms all connected for fast access to patient information.

10. The _____ contains patient and encounter information, often used to correlate the patient to the file identification.

11. A numerical patient record identification system, where the patient is given a new number for each visit, however with each new admission, the previous record is retrieved and filed in the folder with the most recent visit is called _____ numbering.

12. In a _____ system the patient record is filed under the same number for all visits.

13. The filing method of organizing folders in numerical order is _____ filing.

14. A copier-like machine called a _____ is used to convert paper-based records into digital images for a computerized health care record

15. A filing method in which the patient's MR# is separated into sets for filing, the first set of numbers are tertiary, the second set is called secondary, and the last set of numbers are called primary is called _____ filing.

16. A numerical patient record identification system, which gives the patient a new number for each is called _____ numbering.

17. A physical file called an _____ is used to identify an alternate location of a file, in the paper-based health care record system.

## Multiple Choice

1. In the absence of state laws regarding retention of health care records, HCFA requires that records be maintained for:
   A. 10 years
   B. 21 years
   C. 30 years
   D. 5 years

2. To prepare for unexpected events such as a Bomb threat, hurricane, or flood, a facility should routinely exercise which of the policies:
   A. Confidentiality
   B. Release of Information
   C. Disaster Planning
   D. Code Blue

3. Can you identify which of the following is NOT an alphabetic filing rule:
   A. Suffixes are considered after the middle name or initial.
   B. All punctuation and possessives are ignored.
   C. Abbreviations and shortened names are ignored.
   D. Personal names are filed last name, followed by first name, then middle initial.

4. Color coding of the numerical identification on the end tab of a file folder:
   A. Prevents messy files
   B. Aids the identification of misfiles
   C. Is mandatory under JCAHO standards
   D. Warrants approval from the safety committee

5. The machine used to input a paper document into a computerized imaging system is called a
   A. copier
   B. indexer
   C. mapper
   D. scanner

6. Images stored in a document imaging system must be _____ for identification and future retrieval:
   A. copied
   B. indexed
   C. mapped
   D. emailed

7. Which of the following file furniture would not be efficient in a numerical filing system:
   A. file cabinet
   B. open shelves
   C. compressible shelves
   D. microfilm

8. Which of the following methods assist security of records on a computerized system:
   A. microfilm
   B. data dictionary
   C. scanning
   D. routine backups

## Matching

1. _____ computer-based patient records
2. _____ computerized records
3. _____ serial
4. _____ unit
5. _____ serial unit
6. _____ family unit
7. _____ index
8. _____ scanner
9. _____ retention schedule
10. _____ microfilm

A. an alternative method for storing records

B. a file identification system in which the patient receives the same number for all admissions.

C. A file identification system in which the patient receives a new number for each subsequent admission.

D. A file identification system which assigns the same number to an entire family, uniquely identifying each member by a modifier.

E. A file identification system in which the patient receives a new number for each subsequent admission; however, each previous admission is brought forward and filed with the most recent visit.

F. A method of identifying patient records in a computer-based system.

G. The length of time required for maintenance of records.

H. A copier like piece of equipment used to input paper records in a document imaging system.

I. A document imaging system.

J. A system of patient health records which uses a database.

## Critical Thinking Exercises

1.  On a shelf/case that is 36 inches wide with 8 shelves, how many square inches of file space are available?

2.  If you have 12,000 records to file – averaging 2 inches per chart – how many inches of file space do you need? Using the information in Question 1, how many shelves would you need?

3.  The file room in a recently acquired clinic (which filed records alphabetically) must be converted to terminal digit. List the steps involved in the conversion.

4.  Given the file space area of 20 feet × 40 feet with ceiling height of 10 feet (use grid paper, each block equals 1 foot), determine which filing furniture is best to store 40,000 records, average 1 inch thickness. Keep in mind OSHA requirements for aisle and exit space.

## What Else Is Available?

The companion site has links to information about file furniture and equipment, and restoration/preservation of damaged records.

# 6

# Uses of Health Data

## Up to Speed Notes

▶ There are a significant number of ways that health information is used. The uses can be directly related to a health care facility or they may involve national policy, health insurance, or litigation. Can you list the various ways health information is used? If you need assistance, Table 6-1 summarizes the uses of health information.

▶ Accreditation is an important part of the health care facilities business. Various agencies produce standards by which a facility is surveyed to determine whether or not the facility will be granted accreditation. Many of these standards pertain to the documentation and maintenance of health information. Can you describe the type of record review required by JCAHO? Do you know how often the review should be performed? Do you know who is involved in the review?

▶ Health care facilities have numerous committees. These committees meet to perform some of the business required of a health care facility. List the committees who use health information. Can you explain how each committee uses health information?

▶ Like any business, health care facilities are continually trying to improve. "Quality improvement" is the term used to describe this quality effort. There are several QI methods a health care facility can use to improve processes. Can you list and explain two of these methods? How would the health information technologist be involved (directly or indirectly) in each method?

▶ Health Information Management departments routinely receive requests for health information. Using the information learned in this Chapter can you identify three appropriate requests for health information from an entity outside of the health care facility?

▶ Health information is used for patient care. It is used to communicate the patient's progress with the health care professionals involved in the patients care during the patient's stay. Explain how health information is used to improve patient care.

▶ Documentation in the health care record reveals the type of care provided to the patient. Professional associations, accreditation agencies, and the health care facility each have standards that determine how health information is documented. Explain how record reviews are used to evaluate the quality of care provided to patients.

▶ Quality assurance is a retrospective analysis of the functions or processes in a health care department or facility. Prior to the QI effort, JCAHO required facilities to perform a facility-wide process known as the 10-step method. Can you identify the steps in this quality assurance process? If you need help, review Table 6-4.

▶ Numerous regulations and standards govern health information. The state that licenses a health care facility will have regulations regarding health information. The federal government requires specific documentation and maintenance of health information pertaining to Medicare beneficiaries. Accreditation agencies also set standards for health care facilities regarding health information. Given the following standard, explain what is expected of the health information management department. EXAMPLE STANDARD ONLY: Standard HIM 3.4.12: The facility health care delinquent records will not exceed 50% of the average monthly discharge.

## Vocabulary

1. _____ is a quality improvement technique used to solicit participation and information from an entire group.

2. A supervisor and her team of employees are confronted with two solutions to a problem; each solution involves time, money, and space, which quality management tool might the supervisor use to choose a solution: _____.

3. A predetermined course of treatment for a patient with a particular diagnosis is known as a _____.

4. A method used to effectively manage patients during their hospitalization is known as _____.

5. Each month the Tumor Registry personnel are required to report the _____ of breast cancer for the facility. They report this statistic by determining the number of new cases of breast cancer for the month.

6. The method of reviewing patient information during hospitalization is known as _____.

7. The _____ preceded the JCAHO in the survey of hospitals against set standards.

8. Successful completion of a Medicare Conditions of Participation survey results in _____ for the health care facility.

9. To improve quality according to a standard, a health care facility may use _____, the comparison of itself to that of a similar superior performer.

10. _____ is the qualitative review of health care records to determine the appropriateness of care according to the patient's diagnosis.

11. Health information may be used in _____ to support the plaintiff's claim.

12. Thorough review of the patient's health information to determine pertinence, appropriateness, or compliance with standards is _____.

13. _____ refers to death within a population.

14. Health information may be analyzed to support a _____ campaign to promote the facility within its community.

15. Retrospective review of a product of a service is _____.

16. The number of existing cancer cases reported by the tumor registry is known as _____.

17. A quality improvement effort regarding completion of the patient advance directive would require an _____ team.

18. _____ refers to disease within a population.

19. A quality improvement effort regarding scanning of loose reports would require an _____ team.

20. The alternative to quality assurance, _____ is an ongoing effort to improve processes within the health care facility.

21. The _____ process would be initiated following a patient fall from the bed, to gather information and coordinate the claim.

22. The monies collected by the health care facility from the payer is known as _____.

23. Physicians may perform _____ to determine the cause or best treatment for a particular disease.

24. Ensuring appropriate, efficient, and effective patient care is a process of _____.

25. The review of the record performed postdischarge is known as _____.

## Multiple Choice

1. Voluntary accreditation attained by successfully undergoing a survey against the standards set forth in the comprehensive accreditation manual for hospitals is given by
   A. MCOP
   B. HCFA
   C. Medicare
   D. JCAHO

2. Certification may be obtained by complying with which one of the following:
   A. MCOP
   B. MPI
   C. Medicaid billing regulations
   D. JCAHO

3. In the popular PDCA quality improvement method, which step of the process involves monitoring effectiveness of the solution over a period of time?
   A. Plan
   B. DO
   C. Check
   D. Act

4. Which of the following Medical Staff committees reviews medication usage?
   A. Surgical Case review
   B. P & T Committee
   C. Medical Executive Committee
   D. Credentials Committee

5. Which of the following committees acts as a liaison to the Governing board of the facility?
   A. Surgical Case Review
   B. P & T Committee
   C. Medical Executive Committee
   D. Credentials Committee

6. Which of the following is important process in the determination of the facility's compliance with documentation standards?
   A. Physician profile review
   B. Record review
   C. Medication review
   D. PDCA

7. The predecessor of the JCAHO was
   A. Hospital standardization
   B. AHIMA
   C. NCQA
   D. ACS

8. Infections acquired by patients while they are in the hospital are known as:
   A. nosocomial infections
   B. comorbidities
   C. secondary infections
   D. opportunistic infections

9. The committee often responsible for review of health care records according to accreditation standards, physician record completion statistics, and acting as a consultant to the director of health information management is the:
   A. HIM Committee
   B. Safety Committee
   C. Infection Control Committee
   D. P & T Committee

10. The term used to describe the continuous improvement of processes within a facility is:
    A. QA
    B. QM
    C. QI
    D. UM

## Matching

1. _____ Figure 6-12
2. _____ Figure 6-13
3. _____ Figure 6-14
4. _____ Table 6-6
5. _____ Table 6-5

A. Bar chart
B. Survey
C. Line graph
D. Decision matrix
E. Pie chart

## Critical Thinking Exercises

1. Given the following information, create a table and bar chart to represent the percentage of delinquent records for this facility:

   Diamonte Hospital recorded the following delinquent record statistics for last year: January - 200, February - 215, March - 145, April - 197, May - 204, June - 222, July - 208, August - 275, September - 244, October - 231, November - 188, December - 178. The average monthly discharges (AMD) for this facility are 440.

2. Using the Generic Record Review Form, indicate where each criterium will be found in the health care record. You may use the form on the website and create a new column to indicate this information.

3. Using one of the problems listed below, or one that you are familiar with in a Health Information Management department, and identify the members of the QI team to improve the process/problem.

   Backlog of loose report scanning
   Backlog in release of information
   Missing charts, chart locator system is not reliable

## What Else Is Available?

The companion site contains the following additional information:
   Figure 6-08  Generic record review form
   Figure 6-09  Clinical pertinence form
   links to websites:
   www.jcaho.org
   http://www.os.dhhs.gov/
   http://www.carf.org/

# 7

# Retrieval and Reporting of Health Information

## Up to Speed Notes

▶ A patient's health care record from one visit to the health care facility contains an enormous amount of information. In order to quickly analyze and compare health information we capture data elements in the form of a patient abstract. The abstract is a summary of the patient's stay. List 10 elements of a patient abstract. Explain how this information is captured.

▶ A data set is group of elements collected for a specific purpose. A data set is also a standard method for collecting data elements so that they can be compared. In order to compare data we must be sure that everyone is collecting the information the same way. A database is a collection of data. The data collection can occur on paper or in a computer software program. Identify the data set mandated for inpatient discharges, ambulatory care, and long-term care.

▶ The information entered into a computerized abstract creates a database. This database is then used to retrieve patient specific or aggregate data. Explain how a health information technician assures the quality of the health information database.

▶ Many departments in a health care facility need health information to complete their duties, study processes, or monitor productivity. Can you explain two circumstances where a department may request health information or statistics?

▶ Agencies outside of the facility require reporting of health information. Specifically, statistics may be reported to a local or state hospital organization for comparison and monitoring. Additionally, accreditation agencies require reporting of sentinel events. Can you identify the information that must be reported by a health care facility to the Department of Vital Statistics?

▶ Due to the various requests for aggregate and patient-specific health information the health information technologist must know how to retrieve the appropriate data to fulfill the request. Can you explain the difference between aggregate and patient-specific data?

▶ By entering each patient abstract into a computer system a database is created. Health information technologists use this database to gather information or data for analysis or comparison. Can you identify 10 elements of a patient abstract? If you need help refer to figure 7-6.

▶ The health information technologist uses the database created by the patient abstracts to query for reports. Can you explain how this function operates?

▶ Some requests for health information require all of the cases that fit into a specific category. Other requests will ask for a portion of the patients that fit into a category. Can you explain the difference between a population and a sample?

▶ In order to retrieve the appropriate data or information from the database the health information technician must understand all of the data elements contained in the database. The health information database must have a corresponding data dictionary. Explain the purpose of the data dictionary. Identify the best way to find the number of patients discharged in a given month with a specific diagnosis.

▶ There are several different tools used to gather, analyze, and present data for quality improvement. List and explain three data gathering tools, and four data analysis tools.

▶ Health information is often requested in the form of a statistic. Using the table below, compute the following statistics:
Average Length of Stay (ALOS)
Bed Occupancy Rate
Nosocomial Infection Rate

### 1ˢᵀ QUARTER, JANUARY–MARCH 2002
### DIAMONTE HOSPITAL

**INPATIENT SERVICE DAYS**

Adults & Children (A&C) .............................. 4322
Newborns ..................................................... 780

**DISCHARGE DAYS**

Adults & Children (A&C) .............................. 4455
Newborns ..................................................... 785

**BEDS**

Adult & Children (A&C) ................................ 150
Newborn ....................................................... 20

**SURGERY**

Surgical procedures w/ general anesthesia .... 321
Procedures w/ IV conscious sedation ............ 188

**INFECTIONS**

Nosocomial infections ..................................... 24
Post-operative infections ................................ 18

**DISCHARGES**

Adults & Children (A&C) .............................. 1222
Newborns ..................................................... 380

# Vocabulary

1.  The number of patients present in the health care facility, counted at the same time each day, is called the _____.

2.  All of the students registered for this class could be called a _____.

3.  Another name for a data illustration: _____.

4.  The HIM department computer contains a _____.

5.  The subjective portion of a SOAP progress notes is _____ data. Also information obtained by a caregiver after observation of the patient.

6.  Data processed into a meaningful format is known as _____.

7.  An _____ is a summary of the patient record.

8.  UHDDS and UACDS are examples of a _____.

9.  A report of a group of patients including their age is an example of _____ data.

10. Diagnosis, physician, or procedure _____ are used to organize and retrieve specific data from the HIM database.

11. The result of a query is also known as a _____.

12. The Eye, Ear, Nose, and Throat hospital that performs ambulatory surgery must complete the _____ on all of their patients.

13. Analysis, interpretation, and presentation of numbers is called _____.

14. To study only the female students registered for this class is to examine a _____.

15. Diamonte Hospital, an acute care facility, must complete the _____ on all patients discharged from the facility.

16. An organization of data elements in rows and columns is called a _____.

17. When the clerk requests a report from a computer system, they are said to _____ the database.

18. The diagnosis index is an example of _____ data.

19. A database of specific cancer or trauma information is an example of a _____.

## Multiple Choice

1. A federally mandated database collected on all inpatients discharged from a hospital.
   A. MPI
   B. UHDCS
   C. UHDDS
   D. UACDS

2. The CEO requests information on the number of arthroscopies performed annually. What information should be requested from the database to be included on the report?
   A. patient name only
   B. patient name, MR#, ICD-9-CM procedure code, discharge date, surgeon
   C. patient name, procedure description, surgery date
   D. surgeon

3. Identify the request below for aggregate health information
   A. request for report on all DRG 127 for the month of June
   B. request for patient information, MR# 02-34-65, DRG 127
   C. request for 1st case of CHF for the 3rd quarter
   D. request for record of patient # 197808, under the care of Dr. L. Kobob

4. Given a request for the number of medicare CHF cases for the month of April, how would you query the database to sort the report?
   A. patient gender
   B. patient age
   C. financial class
   D. diagnosis

5. The database mandated for collection on outpatients is:
   A. MPI
   B. UHDCS
   C. UHDDS
   D. UACDS

6. Birth certificates, completed by the health care facility, are registered with:
   A. Department of Motor Vehicles
   B. Department of Live Births
   C. Department of Complete Statistics
   D. Department of Vital Records

7. Which of the following graphs would best illustrate the following information: of the 440 discharges for the month of June, 340 were Medicare, 60 were Medicaid, 20 were insurance, 20 were private pay.
   A. pie chart
   B. line chart
   C. brainstorming
   D. decision matrix

8. Identify the statement that best describes the patient abstract.
   A. patient database
   B. summary of the patient's stay
   C. summary of the patient's medical history
   D. patient demographics

9. A sample is a small group within a:
   A. dataset
   B. database
   C. aggregate group
   D. population

10. The patient abstract is an example of:
    A. demographic data
    B. primary data
    C. secondary data
    D. tertiary data

# Matching

Table 7-1 data set by facility type

1. HCFA

2. Primary data

3. UHDDS

4. Statistics

5. UACDS

6. Secondary data

7. RAI

8. table

9. MDS

10. graph

A. The federal agency responsible for Medicare

B. Data arranged in rows and columns

C. An instrument used to evaluate long-term care patients

D. The ALOS for 50% of the chronic obstructive pulmonary disease (COPD) patients is 8 days

E. A data set for ambulatory care patients

F. representation of numbers on a bar chart

G. A data set for inpatients

H. Information taken directly from the patient

I. A data set for long-term care patients

J. Reports queried from the health information database

## Critical Thinking Exercises

1. Using the form on the website and the following scenario, complete the Birth Certificate for Baby Girl Smith.

   Just as her parents before her, Baby girl Luke was born Friday May 18, 2002 after a lengthy labor, at 2:30am at Diamonte Hospital. Although at first things were tense in the delivery room (Apgar at 1 minute = 5, Apgar at 5 minutes = 9), Tina finally heard her baby cry approximately 5 minutes following the birth. Tina's obstetrician, Dr. Vongeaux, congratulated Tina and assured her that everything appeared normal.

   Out of respect to her grandmother, the baby's mother Tina Marie (D.O.B. 11/30/72), decided to name her: Grace Catherine. The father, Christian David (D.O.B. 06/16/70), out of town on business, missed the birth of his daughter.

2. Using the form on the website and the following scenario, complete the Death Certificate.

   Documented by Nurse Harold Glenn; Diamonte Hospital, March 11, 2001, 10:33 pm. Following surgery for GSW to the Right upper quadrant, RUQ, John Thomas Rocke was pronounced dead by his internal medicine physician, Terrence Ford, M.D.

3. Using the Discharge summary on the website and the paper abstract form (text Figure 7-6), complete a patient abstract.

## What Else Is Available?

The companion site also has:

   Birth Certificate
   Death Certificate
   Patient Discharge Summary and abstract form Figure 7-6.

# *8*

# Confidentiality and Compliance

## Up to Speed Notes

- ▶ Consent is also required in order to treat a patient. Explain informed consent. List three ways that a patient can consent to medical treatment.
- ▶ Health care facilities can be both licensed and accredited. Explain the difference between licensure and accreditation.
- ▶ In general, release of patient-specific information requires the consent of the patient. List three ways that a patient can consent to release of information.
- ▶ In some circumstances, patient-specific information can be released without the consent of the patient. List three reasons that information can be released without patient consent.
- ▶ Jurisdiction refers to the authority of a particular court to decide a particular case. A court may have jurisdiction over the issue and/or the persons involved, for example. List examples of issues over which municipal, state, and federal courts may have jurisdiction.
- ▶ Some health records are considered 'sensitive' and should be managed carefully. List two types of 'sensitive' records. Describe what type(s) of additional controls should be in place to manage these records.
- ▶ Some requests for release of information require special consent. List the medical conditions that require special consent for release of information. Identify the difference(s) between a basic consent for release of information and a special consent.
- ▶ There are specific steps that must be taken in order to satisfy a request for release of a copy of all or part of a record. List these steps and describe why they are important.
- ▶ There are two specific types of subpoenas discussed in this chapter. Name them and explain their use.

# Vocabulary

1. A permission that is given after the event to which the permission applies is _____.

2. Health information must not be disclosed inappropriately, because it is _____.

3. Health records can be used as evidence in a court of law, because of the _____.

4. If a facility meets the standards set by a licensing or accrediting body, it is said to be in _____.

5. In order for a court to hear a case, the court must have _____ over the issue or the parties.

6. _____ is a permission given by a competent individual, of legal age, with full knowledge or understanding of the risks, potential benefits, and potential consequences of the permission.

7. Operational or procedural services that are provided by individuals or organizations who are not employees of the facility for which the services are being provided are said to have been _____.

8. Permission to perform a medical procedure or to release information generally requires the patient's _____.

9. Prospective consent for treatment is contained in the _____.

10. The ability to retrieve health information and provide it to requestors refers to _____.

11. The _____ prohibits most testimony by parties not directly involved in the event.

12. The legal foundation for confidentiality is _____.

13. The party who initiates litigation is the _____.

14. The _____ brings a lawsuit against the _____.

15. The process of engaging in the legal proceedings of a lawsuit is _____.

# Multiple Choice

1. All of the following are elements of the Business Record Rule EXCEPT:
   A. Documentation is contemporaneous with the events it describes
   B. Records are maintained in the normal course of business
   C. Records are kept in accordance with JCAHO standards
   D. Documentation is recorded by those who are in a position to know the facts of the events they describe

2. Conditions of Admission are an example of:
   A. Prospective consent
   B. Retrospective consent
   C. Access
   D. Jurisdiction

3. Federal court may have jurisdiction over all of the following EXCEPT:
   A. Cases involving citizens of different States
   B. Questions of treaty
   C. Litigation involving events occurring on federal land
   D. Amounts over $10,000

4. The practice of maintaining confidentiality in healthcare is based on:
   A. Prospective consent
   B. Retrospective consent
   C. Physician-patient privilege
   D. Attorney-client privilege

5. The new nursing supervisor is discussing with you her plans for the unit. She wants to hang a board on the wall of the nursing unit listing each patient's name, room number, working diagnosis, and medication schedule. You advise her that:
   A. This is a good idea, since it will facilitate coordination of care
   B. This is a violation of confidentiality to display patient-specific information in a public place
   C. This is not a good idea, because it is a violation of prospective consent
   D. The physicians won't like it, because it will show everyone who has the most patients

6. An insurance company may obtain patient records by all of the following EXCEPT:
   A. Prospective consent under the Conditions of Admission
   B. Automatically, under 42CFR
   C. Prospective consent obtained when the patient became insured
   D. Retrospective consent obtained after the patient is discharged

7. A patient presents in the HIM Department requesting a copy of the record for his recent appendectomy. Upon inquiry, the patient reveals that, in addition to wanting a record of the operation, he had an allergic reaction to the anesthesia and wants to keep a record of this event in order to avoid a similar problem in the future. The patient should be advised to request a copy of:
   A. The entire record
   B. The Operative Report

C. The Operative Report and the Anesthesia Records

D. The Discharge Summary

8. Your facility charges a $10 search fee plus $1.00 per page to copy records up to 100 pages. All pages in excess of 100 are charged $.50 per page. Based on this schedule, what is the fee for a 125-page record?

   A. $112.50

   B. $122.50

   C. $125

   D. $135

9. The purpose of the JCAHO Steering Committee is to:

   A. Ensure that compliance with current standards is evaluated

   B. Conduct mock surveys

   C. Prepare staff for the JCAHO visit

   D. All of the above

10. A valid consent for release of information contains all of the following EXCEPT:

   A. Patient's name

   B. Patient's marital status

   C. Patient's date of birth

   D. Date of the request

11. A 16-year-old patient presents in the emergency room for treatment of stomach pain. She is conscious, alert, and oriented. Of the following, who is the appropriate individual to sign the consent for treatment?

   A. The patient

   B. The patient's mother

   C. The patient's husband

   D. No consent is necessary for this emergency treatment

## Matching

Number the steps in a civil lawsuit in their correct order:

1. Appeal

2. Complaint

3. Discovery

4. Pre-trial conference

5. Satisfying the judgment

6. Trial

## Critical Thinking Exercises

1. The federal government passed the Health Insurance Portability and Accountability Act in 1996. This legislation has an impact on implementation of an electronic patient record as well as on confidentiality and privacy. Follow the links on the companion site to find out the latest information about this important legislation. How do the associated privacy regulations impact what you learned in this Chapter about consents?

2. What internal control function(s) is/are performed by the HIM department in providing access to health information?

3. List the steps in processing a request for a copy of a health record. Based on your list, write a procedure to instruct clerical staff to perform this task. Be sure to include all of the tools that the employee will require as well as what to do if there is a problem. If you are unsure how to proceed, refer to Chapter Ten in the text.

4. The release of information function is one of the most common functions in an HIM department to be outsourced. If you were the supervisor of this area, what would be your biggest concerns in outsourcing the function?

5. A patient has been admitted to your facility for treatment of pneumonia. He gave insurance information to the patient registration department. During the course of treatment, the patient is found to have AIDS. After discharge, the patient's insurance company asks for a copy of the record. Can the insurance company obtain the record at this point? What are the issues?

6. A married woman was admitted to the acute care facility for the purpose of childbirth. She had insurance coverage from her employment and gave patient registration that information. That evening, she gave birth to a boy and went home with her husband and the baby the next day. She named her husband as the baby's father for the birth certificate. Two months later, the husband presented in the HIM department to obtain a copy of the baby's birth record to take to their new pediatrician. Should he be given a copy of the record? What are the issues?

7. What impact does an electronic patient record have on the release-of-information function?

## What Else Is Available?

The companion site contains links to government and other web sites that detail and explain the Health Insurance Portability and Accountability Act and the regulations that have been published to enforce it.

# 9

# Reimbursement

## Up to Speed Notes

▶ The payment for healthcare services is usually referred to as reimbursement. List the four types of reimbursement.

▶ Each type of reimbursement has unique characteristics and a different approach to risk. Compare and contrast the four types of reimbursement, identifying the financial risk to the parties involved.

▶ HCFAs success with using DRGs as the basis for reimbursement has prompted the development of other, similar systems. List the other systems discussed in the chapter. What health care environments are reimbursed using these methods?

▶ Health care insurance involves the assumption of the risk of financial loss by a party other than the patient. Describe how insurance companies can afford to assume such risk.

▶ The text discussed three different types of health insurance. List them and describe why they are different.

▶ The federal government funds health care reimbursement at many different levels. Describe the federal government involvement in health care reimbursement. What government agencies are involved in this process?

▶ Billing for physician services is accomplished using the HCFA 1500 billing form. What data is required on this form?

▶ Hospital-based services are billed using the UB-92. What data is required on this form?

▶ Identify and describe the players in reimbursement.

▶ Identify unethical billing practices.

# Vocabulary

1. A data collection device that facilitates the accurate capture of ambulatory care diagnoses and services is an _____.

2. A health care provider applies to a payer for reimbursement by submitting a _____.

3. A savings account in which health care and certain child-care costs can be set aside and paid using pre-tax funds is a _____.

4. Before a payer reimburses for a claim, there may be an amount for which the patient is personally responsible, called a _____.

5. Fees or costs are also called _____.

6. HCFAs prospective payment system for hospital-based ambulatory care is based on _____.

7. ICD-9-CM diagnosis and procedures codes are used to derive the DRG by following the flowchart in a _____.

8. ICD-9-CM is coordinated and maintained by a group of four organizations collectively called the _____.

9. In Long-Term Care, the _____ is used to determine the prospective payment.

10. In order to standardize and facilitate accurate billing, health care facilities maintain a database of all potential services to a patient called a _____.

11. In return for the payment of a premium an _____ assumes the risk of paying some or all of the cost of providing health care services to an individual or group of individuals.

12. Medicare uses _____ to process its claims and reimbursements.

13. Procedures and controls to ensure correct coding are part of a _____.

14. Prospective payment for acute care is based on _____.

15. Reimbursement to a health care provider on a per-patient basis is _____.

16. The amount paid to an insurance company by or on behalf of the insured is called a _____.

17. The process of determining the most accurate DRG payment is _____.

18. The process of submitting claims or rendering invoices is called _____.

19. The systematic collection of specific charges for services rendered to a patient is called _____.

## Multiple Choice

1. The payer had an agreement with the physician to pay the 'usual and customary fee', less 10%. This is an example of:
   A. Prospective Payment
   B. Fee-for-service
   C. Discounted fee-for-service
   D. Capitation

**USE THE FOLLOWING SCENARIO TO ANSWER QUESTIONS 2 AND 3:**

The 82-year-old patient presented in the physician's office for a routine physical examination. He gave the receptionist two cards, evidencing his primary, government-funded insurance plan that pays for most of the bill and an additional, private plan that covers the remaining charges.

2. The patient's primary insurance is most likely:
   A. Discounted fee-for-service
   B. Wraparound plan
   C. Medicare
   D. Capitation

3. The patient's secondary insurance is called:
   A. Discounted fee-for-service
   B. Wraparound plan
   C. Medicare
   D. Capitation

4. The physician charged the patient $75 for the office visit. The patient paid the physician $5 and the patient's insurance company paid the physician $70. This method of reimbursement is called:
   A. Discounted fee-for-service
   B. Wraparound plan
   C. Fee-for-service
   D. Co-payment

5. The physician charged the patient $75 for the office visit. The patient paid the physician $5 and the patient's insurance company paid the physician $70. The patient's portion of the payment is called:
   A. Discounted fee-for-service
   B. Wraparound plan
   C. Fee-for service
   D. Co-payment

6. Title XVIII is the amendment to the Social Security Act that established:
   A. Medicare
   B. Medicaid
   C. Capitation
   D. The Prospective Payment System

7. The payment rate established by an insurance company, based on its knowledge of the regional charges for a service are called:
   A. Discounted fee-for-service
   B. Fee-for-service
   C. Usual and customary charges
   D. Capitation

8. Unlike prospective payment for acute care, long-term care prospective payment is on what basis?
   A. Lump-sum
   B. Capitation
   C. Per Diem
   D. Discounted fee-for-service

9. An organization which insures as well as owns or exerts employer control over the health care providers is a(n):
   A. Health Maintenance Organization
   B. Preferred Provider Organization
   C. Indemnity Company
   D. Blue Cross Organization

10. The department in a hospital that is primarily responsible for submitting bills or claims for reimbursement is:
    A. Health Information Management
    B. Utilization Review
    C. Patient Registration
    D. Patient Accounts

# Matching

Match the definition on the left with the health insurance terminology on the right.

1. Amount of cost that the beneficiary must incur before the insurance will assume liability for the remaining cost
2. Contractor that manages the health care claims
3. One who is eligible to receive or is receiving benefits from an insurance policy or a managed care program
4. Party who is financially responsible for reimbursement of health care cost
5. Payer's payment for specific health care services or, in managed care, the health care services that will be provided or for which the provider will be paid
6. Payment by a third party to a provider of health care
7. Request for payment by the insured or the provider for services covered

A. Beneficiary
B. Benefit
C. Claim
D. Deductible
E. Fiscal intermediary
F. Payer
G. Reimbursement

## Critical Thinking Exercises

1. Insurance coverage is an important employee benefit, because it is so expensive. The example in your text, Figure 9-1, uses $5,000 per year as the premium for all of the insured parties. Is that a realistic premium? Try contacting an insurance company in your area to see what it would cost you to purchase basic health insurance. Some companies will allow you to inquire via their websites. Look at the difference between an indemnity contract and a managed care contract. If you were a company with 500 employees, how much would health insurance cost per year, based on your research?

2. Why isn't long-term care reimbursement based on DRGs? You can obtain a copy of the MDS from the HCFA website. Compare and contrast this data set with the UHDDS. Why do you think it is so different?

3. The Proposed Rules for Prospective Payment for Inpatient Rehabilitation were published in November 2000. Would you expect them to be more like acute care or long-term care? Check the HCFA website to locate these rules. What is the status of these rules? How is outpatient rehabilitation reimbursed?

4. Physician services are reimbursed under the Resource-Based Relative Value System (RBRVS). This is a set of predetermined charges for specific physician services. What can you find about this system on the HCFA website? What type of reimbursement system is this?

5. How does case mix analysis help health care providers plan for the future?

## What Else Is Available?

The companion site contains links to government and insurance company web sites.

# 10

# Human Resource Management

## Up to Speed Notes

- Although there are many different types and sizes of health care facilities, the functions and responsibilities of Health Information Management Departments are essentially the same. Identify the basic functions of an HIM department.
- While the functions and responsibilities of HIM departments remain essentially the same, the manner or order in which the functions are performed varies with each facility. Explain how the functions listed above are organized within the HIM department. Express the workflow in the form of a flow chart.
- Depending upon the size of the HIM department, there may be one person performing each function or several employees performing one function. As the HIM manager, explain how you will determine the job responsibilities or tasks for each employee.
- Once you have determined the responsibilities and tasks associated with an employees job, it is possible to create a job description. Identify the elements of a job description. Explain performance standards and their relationship to the job description.
- The priorities of an HIM department are often determined by the goals and objectives. Explain these terms and give examples of each.
- There are many responsibilities associated with management of an HIM department. Explain how delegating can improve a manager's effectiveness.
- An important responsibility of management involves the appropriate design of the work environment. You want employees to be comfortable as well as free from potential injury while performing their responsibilities and tasks. Explain and give examples of an ergonomically sound work environment for HIM personnel.
- Appropriate work space design will help employees perform their tasks in a safe, efficient, and effective manner. In a new or renovated HIM department there are some very important areas that should be addressed. Identify the OSHA requirements for file area aisles and exits. Discuss special considerations for design of a transcription area. Finally, identify equipment and supply needs for HIM department functions and services.

- In order to communicate the expectations of management (the employer) to the employee, there are often many rules, policies, and procedures established. Explain and give examples of HIM department rules and policies for employee operations and conduct.

- An important part of management is the supervision (controlling) of the department functions and services. Standards must be established to monitor the functions and services. When a standard is established correctly, with the goals of the department in mind, it will promote effective HIM operations and services. Explain how a standard can be established for one of the basic HIM functions or services.

- Once standards have been established, the work performance of the employees must be monitored. Explain how information is collected to determine whether or not the standards are being met. What happens if the standards are not met consistently? What should happen if the standards are consistently exceeded?

- Employees in the HIM department need equipment and supplies to perform their daily tasks. Faulty equipment and lack of supplies can hinder productivity and cause serious problems in the effectiveness of the HIM department. Explain the standard equipment found in a HIM department. Identify what can be done to assure that supplies do not run out.

- All of the important aspects of an HIM department should be documented in policy and procedure format. Define policy and procedure and provide five (5) example policies for HIM functions and services.

## Vocabulary

1. An _____ works 32-40 hours each week excluding overtime, earning full benefits as offered by the health care facility.

2. The _____ is an illustration used to describe the relationship between departments, positions, and functions within an organization.

3. A formal list of the employee's responsibilities associated with their job is called a _____ .

4. For the 2001-2002 fiscal year the manager has set a _____ to implement a document imaging system.

5. _____ are set guidelines explaining how much work an employee must complete.

6. In order to reach a desired goal the department must establish _____ , directions for achieving a goal.

7. As the new supervisor over the file area, release of Information and Assembly and Analysis, Sandra feels overwhelmed by the number of projects needing her attention. One way that Sandra may relieve the pressure from these projects is to _____ some of the projects to her employees.

8. A _____ involves the review of a function to determine all of the tasks or components that make up an employee's job.

9. It is the responsibility of the employer to provide a safe work environment for the employee to perform his/her job function. One way that this can be accomplished is through design of an _____ work space.

10. The purpose of the organization documented in a formal statement is known as the _____ .

11. The following is _____ of Diamonte Hospital, an equal opportunity employer. All new hires will be drug tested.

12. In the HIM department Judy, the Physician Record Clerk is responsible to Deenie the supervisor and Michelle the Director. This violates the _____ principle.

13. _____ is the amount of work produced by an employee in a given time frame.

14. A process that describes how to comply with a policy is a _____ .

15. Above and beyond the mission statement, a _____ sets a direction for the organization for the future.

16. Janet is a supervisor responsible for 8 coding employees, this statement represents Janet's _____ .

## Multiple Choice

1.  An employee who works 16 - 20 hours each week, occasionally earning partial benefits is:
    A.  FTE
    B.  PRN
    C.  Part time
    D.  LPN

2.  In an organization chart boxes indicate
    A.  line responsibility
    B.  authority
    C.  responsibility
    D.  departments or positions

3.  The HIM Director establish the following: "The HIM department delinquency % will not exceed 50% of AMD by July 1". This is an example of a(n):
    A.  plan
    B.  goal
    C.  objective
    D.  mission

4.  In addition the Director stated, the Suspension procedure will be performed weekly (as approved in the bylaws). This is an example of a(n):
    A.  plan
    B.  goal
    C.  objective
    D.  mission

5.  Broken lines on an organization chart indicate
    A.  line responsibility
    B.  authority
    C.  indirect or shared responsibility
    D.  departments or positions

6.  The governing body
    A.  has the authority to grant privileges to members of the medical staff
    B.  is responsible for quality services provided by the facility
    C.  both A & B
    D.  none of the above

7.  The amount of work in the HIM department is determined by
    A.  the CEO
    B.  the department director
    C.  admissions
    D.  the number of discharges, patient type and length of stay

8. Policy and Procedures should be updated
   A. annually and as needed due to change
   B. only as needed due to change
   C. by the CEO
   D. by the nursing administrator

9. Performance standards measure
   A. quantity
   B. quality
   C. A & B
   D. number of employees

10. Which of the following Fair Employment Laws prohibit discrimination based on race, color, religion or sex?
    A. Fair Labor Standards Act
    B. Civil Rights Act
    C. Americans with Disabilities Act
    D. Age Discrimination in Employment Act

## Matching

1. _____ Concurrent Processing
2. _____ Retrospective Processing
3. _____ PRN
4. _____ FTE
5. _____ Civil Rights Act
6. _____ Fair Labor Standards Act
7. _____ CPT Assistant
8. _____ Coding Clinic

A. A pool of employees used as needed when work load increases.
B. A monthly newsletter published by AHA for outpatient coders.
C. Set minimum wage, overtime pay, and equal pay, child labor, and record keeping requirements for employers.
D. Processing of health care records postdischarge.
E. Quarterly newsletter published by AHA for inpatient coders.
F. HIM functions performed on health care records during the patients stay.
G. an employee who works 32-40 per week earning full benefits.
H. Ensures equal employment opportunity.

## Critical Thinking Exercises

1. Explain the employee evaluation process.

2. Create an advertisement for an open position in an HIM department.

3. Complete the employment application found in the text and on the website.

4. Create a list of questions you might ask an applicant during an interview for a HIM department position.

5. Using the job description Figures 10-8, 10-8a, create performance standards for this position. Try to incorporate these two documents into one.

## What Else Is Available?

Figure 10 - 10, 10-10a, 10-10b, 10-10c; Figure 10-8, 10-8a.

# 11

# Training and Development

## Up to Speed Notes

- New employees must be oriented to the organization and the job during the first few days of employment. List the topics covered during the organization orientation. Then list the topics covered during the HIM department orientation.
- Members of the medical staff and other facility personnel also need to be oriented to the HIM department. Identify topics covered with the Medical Staff. Identify topics covered with other facility personnel.
- Throughout employment there are new processes, changes, and important procedures that must be communicated to the employees so that they understand what is expected. Identify three in-service topics for HIM personnel. Discuss the development an in-service topic for presentation. Remember to consider the issues associated with preparing a training program: assessment of education needs, audience, format, and environment.
- HIM department employees are in constant need of continuing education. Identify specific continuing education needs for the following HIM employees: credentialed employees, coding employees, release of information.
- One of the most important and unified methods of communication to all department employees is the monthly HIM department meeting. During this meeting the director can communicate one message to all employees and document that the information has been discussed. Organize an agenda for HIM department meetings. Using the agenda set up a format for the minutes that must be taken during this meeting. Include a list of all materials that must be kept to document the meeting.
- In lieu of department meetings, managers and employees often use memos to expedite communication or information. Create a memo to the medical staff regarding the new dictation equipment installed for their convenience in the Physician's Lounge.

## Vocabulary

1. _____ indicate a person's specific professional qualifications.

2. The period of time, also known as a grace period, given to a new employee to learn the job and reach the performance standards associated with that job is known as the _____ .

3. _____ are used to record the events, topics, and discussions of a meeting.

4. A name for the training provided to employees of an organization is _____ .

5. A general term for education, instruction, or demonstration of how to perform a job is known as _____ .

6. The term used to describe a training to familiarize a new employee to the job is _____ .

7. An _____ is used to organize the topics to be discussed during a meeting.

8. A written/typed communication tool used to communicate or provide information to members of an organization is a _____ .

9. _____ may be required after attaining a position, credential, or degree intended to keep those persons knowledgeable in core content areas.

## Multiple Choice

1. To make an employee familiar with his/her job and new surroundings the employee must attend
   A. training
   B. orientation
   C. in-service
   D. department meeting

2. The "R" in the common safety acronym RACE used to describe the employees expected response to a fire means
   A. Red
   B. Run
   C. Rescue
   D. Reassure

3. Which of the following organization orientation topics may be presented by an HIM employee
   A. Safety
   B. Infection Control
   C. Personnel Issues
   D. Confidentiality

4. The first step in planning a training, in-service, or continuing education program is
   A. Assessment of education needs
   B. Audience
   C. Area
   D. Inventory of skills

5. Continuing education is critical for coding employees. Which of the following dates is critical in the education of inpatient coders?
   A. January 1
   B. October 1
   C. December 1
   D. July 1

6. To maintain the RHIT credential, the professional must maintain
   A. 20 hours of continuing education each year
   B. 30 hours of continuing education each year
   C. 20 hours of continuing education during a two year cycle
   D. 30 hours of continuing education during a two year cycle

7. A popular form of electronic communication is the
   A. memo
   B. email
   C. fax machine
   D. telephone

8. The first item on the monthly HIM department meeting agenda is
   A. Call to Order
   B. Review of Old Business
   C. New Business
   D. Adjournment

## Matching

1. _____ Training
2. _____ Development
3. _____ Clinical Data Management
4. _____ Code Black
5. _____ Code Pink

A. ongoing improvement of staff personally and professionally.
B. bomb threat
C. orientation, education, and practical experience for a position or job function
D. RHIT core content area
E. infant abduction

## Critical Thinking Exercises

1. Design an education program for the public.

2. Complete a function request form to reserve equipment and space to hold a training program.

3. Discuss the tools used to perform an in-service for coding.

4. Discuss the tools used to perform an in-service for release of information.

## What Else Is Available?

The companion site has links to:

Popular community awareness topics for public education
Function request form

# Answers
# Section

# 1

## Health Care Delivery Systems
### ANSWERS

## Vocabulary

1. "Diabetes" is an example of a **Diagnosis**.

2. A health care organization that has permanent facilities, 24-hour nursing care, and an organized medical staff is a type of **Hospital**.

3. A hospital with an average length of stay less than 30 days, an emergency department, operating suite, and clinical departments to handle a broad range of diagnoses and treatments is most likely an **Acute care facility**.

4. A specialty inpatient facility that focuses on the treatment of individuals who are not adults is a **Children's hospital**.

5. An **Integrated delivery system** provides care to patients at all or most points along the continuum of care.

6. Care for the terminally ill is the focus of **Hospice** care.

7. Health care professionals must adhere to their discipline's **Code of Ethics**.

8. **Home health care** focuses on treating patients where they reside.

9. Medicare waives compliance audits for appropriately accredited facilities by granting them **Deemed status**.

10. Occupational therapy is an example of an **Allied health professional**.

11. Patients whose care requires them to remain in the hospital overnight are called **Inpatients**.

12. The actual number beds that a hospital has available for inpatients is called the **Bed count**.

13. The broad range of services that may be required by a patient in his/her lifetime is referred to as the **Continuum of care**.

14. Voluntary compliance with a set of standards developed by an independent agency is part of the **Accreditation** process.

15. When one physician asks another physician for an opinion regarding the care of a patient, the first physician is asking for a **Consultation**.

## Multiple Choice

1. A patient was admitted to the hospital on September 13 and discharged on September 30. What is the length of stay?

   B. 17 days      30 – 13 = 17

2. A patient was admitted to the hospital on August 20 and discharged on October 6. What is the length of stay?

   A. 47 days      12 days in August, 30 days in September, 5 days in October
   47 days (remember to count the day of admission, but not the day of discharge.)

3. The Community Care Center has 200 beds. It has an average length of stay of 2 years. Most of the patients are elderly, but there are some younger patients with serious chronic illnesses. Community Care Center is most likely a(n):

   C. Long-term care facility

4. Another term for a Consultation is a(n):

   B. Referral

5. Chapone Health Care is an organization that owns a number of different health care facilities: three acute care hospitals, two long-term care facilities, and a number of physician offices. Chapone also owns a rehabilitation hospital and an assisted living facility, which also delivers home care. They deliver care to patients at every point along the continuum of care. Chapone Health Care can be described as a(n):

   D. Integrated Health Care Delivery System

6. The following patients were discharged from pediatrics for the week 7/16/01 – 7/22/01:

   | Patient Name | Admission Date | Discharge Date |
   | --- | --- | --- |
   | Groot | 7/13/01 | 7/15/01 |
   | Smith | 7/12/01 | 7/15/01 |
   | Brown | 7/11/01 | 7/16/01 |
   | Kowalski | 7/10/01 | 7/20/01 |
   | Zhong | 7/09/01 | 7/19/01 |
   | Frank | 6/29/01 | 7/18/01 |

   Total length of stay of all patients: 49 days      Average length of stay of 7 patients:
   49 divided by 7 = 7 days

   The average length of stay of these patients is:

   B. 7 days

7. Which of the following is NOT an agency within the Department of Health and Human Services?

   D. OSHA

8. Medicare is administered by:

   B. HCFA

9. A facility which focuses totally on palliative care is a(n):

   B. Hospice

10. Which of the following is an example of a diagnosis?
    A. Tonsillitis

11. Which of the following is an example of a procedure?
    C. Tonsillectomy

12. Which of the following qualifies an acute care facility for 'deemed status'?
    C. JCAHO accreditation

## Matching

Match the diagnosis, activity, or patient group on the left with the name of the specialty on the right.

| | |
|---|---|
| 1. B | 8. F |
| 2. J | 9. C |
| 3. G | 10. L |
| 4. I | 11. D |
| 5. N | 12. O |
| 6. E | 13. K |
| 7. H | 14. A |
| | 15. M |

Match accrediting bodies on the left with the type of organization on the right. Some accrediting bodies accredit more than one type of organization.

1. B
2. E
3. F
4. B
5. A, B, C, E, F
6. D

# 2

## Data Elements

## *ANSWERS*

## Vocabulary

1.  A single letter, number, or symbol is a **character**.

2.  The study of disease trends and occurrences is **epidemiology**.

3.  The quality that data reflects the known or acceptable range of values for the specific data is called **data validity**.

4.  The quality of data being correct is called **accuracy**.

5.  A collection or series of related characters is a **field**.

6.  Data collected for the purpose of patient identification is **demographic data**.

7.  Data collected during the investigation of the patient's current health situation is called **clinical data**.

8.  In a database, a list of details about each field is a **data dictionary**.

9.  The smallest element or unit of knowledge is **data**.

10. After all other payment sources are exhausted, the **guarantor** is responsible for the remaining balance of payments.

11. The initial collection of height, weight, temperature, and blood pressure on a patient's first visit to a physician is called **baseline** data.

12. Data which pertain to the patient's personal life and personal habits, such as marital status and religion, are **socioeconomic data**.

13. Data collected about the party who will pay for the patient's health care is **financial data**.

## Multiple Choice

1. Which of the following is a symptom?
   C. Runny nose

2. The ability of a patient to see a physician without an appointment is called:
   B. Open-access

3. Which of the following is an example of demographic data?
   A. Address

4. Another term for a Demographic data is:
   D. Indicative

5. Of the following workers in a physician's office, who is the most likely one to collect the patient's blood pressure?
   B. Nurse

6. Which of the following is NOT an example of clinical data?
   B. Smokes 2 packs of cigarettes daily

7. If a patient's insurance company has reimbursed the physician for the appropriate amount and there is still a balance due in the patient's account, the physician must apply next for payment to the:
   A. Guarantor

8. Which of the following is an example of a field?
   D. All of the above

**USE THE SAMPLE DATA DICTIONARY BELOW TO ANSWER QUESTIONS 9 - 10**

| Name | Definition | Size | Type | Example |
|------|-----------|------|------|---------|
| FNAME | Patient's First Name | 15 Characters | Alphabetic | Jane |
| LNAME | Patient's Last Name | 15 Characters | Alphabetic | Jones |
| HTEL | Patient's Home Telephone Number | 12 Characters | Alpha-numeric | 973-555-3331 |
| TEMP | Patient's Temperature | 5 Characters | Numeric | 98.6 |

9. Using 12 alpha-numeric characters is one way to capture the patient's home telephone number. List at least one other way to capture that data.
   3 fields: area code, exchange, number
   2 fields: area code, exchange+number
   1 field: 10-digits, recorded as a numeric field

10. List and describe two additional fields that would be needed to capture a patient's entire name.
    Title (Mr., Mrs., Miss, Ms., Dr.)
    Middle Name (either initial or entire name)
    Courtesy designations (Esq., OSM)

11. Using the format above, define the fields that would be needed to capture a patient's diagnosis and a procedure. Refer to Chapter One for examples that you can use.

| Name | Definition | Size | Type | Example |
|------|-----------|------|------|---------|
| DX | Diagnosis | 15 Characters | Alphabetic | Appendicitis |
| PX | Procedure | 15 Characters | Alphabetic | Appendectomy |

## Matching

Match the physician office activity described on the left with the name of the professional most likely to perform it on the right.

1. E

2. C

3. D

4. A

5. B

# 3

## Organization of Data Elements in a Health Record

## *ANSWERS*

### Vocabulary

1. A physician who only performs operations is a **surgeon**.

2. Another was to refer to a form is as a **data collection device**.

3. Another word for therapy is **treatment**.

4. At the end of a hospital stay, a **discharge summary** is usually required to be completed, often as a dictated and transcribed report.

5. If a health care professional is working under the supervision of another, such as a resident being supervised by an attending physician, then the notes written by that professional must be **countersigned** by the supervisor.

6. In medical decision making, the physician's evaluation of the subjective and objective evidence is called the **assessment**.

7. In order to **authenticate** a document other data collection device, a physician may sign the document or enter a password.

8. Routine documentation of the nurse's interaction with a patient is recorded in the **nursing progress notes**.

9. Sometimes a physician needs to ask another physician for an opinion regarding the care of a patient. The physician whom he asks is referred to as the **consultant**.

10. The act of rendering an opinion about another physician's patient is called a **consultation**.

11. The cause or source of a patient's condition or disease is called the **etiology**.

12. The first page in a paper record is usually the **face sheet**.

13. The physician who is primarily responsible for coordinating the care of the patient in the hospital is the **attending physician**.

14. When a patient is first seen by a physician in any health care setting, the physician generally records the patient's chief complaint, pertinent family and social data, and a review of the patient's body systems. This record is called the history.

15. When paper records are organized in chronological order, they are described as: date-oriented, sequential, or integrated records.

## Multiple Choice

1. Which of the following is an element of an acute care admission record?

   C. Name of patient's employer

2. Which of the following data elements is NOT likely to appear on an acute care admission record?

   D. Tobacco use by the patient

3. If a hospital wanted to correspond with a patient after discharge, the appropriate source of the patient's current address would be the:

   D. Latest admission record

4. Which of the following is not a necessary part of a medication record?

   A. Physician's signature

5. Which of the following is an example of the 'P' in SOAP?

   D. Schedule barium swallow.

6. Which of the following is an example of the 'O' in SOAP?

   C. Patient's abdomen is tender to palpation in the epigastric region.

7. The nursing department in your facility has submitted a form to the forms committee for approval. The form is printed on dark gold paper so that it will stand out in the chart. You recommend a light yellow paper instead, because it photocopies better than dark gold. This is an example of taking into consideration:

   B. The needs of all users of the device

8. The purpose of instructions on a data collection device is to:

   C. Help ensure the consistency of data collection

9. All of the following are elements of the UHDDS EXCEPT:

   E. Marital Status

10. When entering physician orders in a computer-based system, the computer can check the authentication to ensure that the individual who entered the data is authorized to do so (that is, that the authentication is correct). This is an example of a computer being used to ensure data:

    A. Validity

## Matching

Match the physician progress note entry on the left with the SOAP note component on the right.

| | |
|---|---|
| 1. D | 3. A |
| 2. C | 4. B |

Match the chart description on the left with the record order on the right.

| | |
|---|---|
| 1. C | 3. B |
| 2. D | 4. A |

Match the definition on the left with the vocabulary word(s) on the right.

| | |
|---|---|
| 1. L | 8. G |
| 2. A | 9. E |
| 3. J | 10. F |
| 4. D | 11. I |
| 5. B | 12. H |
| 6. H | 13. K |
| 7. C | |

# Postdischarge Processing
## *ANSWERS*

## Vocabulary

1. A computer can create a log of processing and access activities called an **audit trail**.

2. A detective control function designed to identify incomplete data in a record is **quantitative analysis**.

3. A list of deficient or other problem data, usually generated by a computer, is an **exception report**.

4. A list of potentially inaccurate or problem data, usually generated by a computer, is an **error report**.

5. A paper record must be **assembled** before it can be analyzed.

6. Another word for an Incomplete System is a **Deficiency System**.

7. Assignment of ICD-9-CM codes to clinical data while the patient is still being treated is **concurrent coding**.

8. Clinicians can evidence supervision of subordinate personnel by **countersigning** the subordinates' documentation.

9. Data that has been obtained, recorded, and/or reported within a pre-determined period satisfies the data quality characteristic of **timeliness**.

10. In a paper record environment, **universal chart order** refers to the maintenance of the same page order both pre- and postdischarge.

11. Parts of paper records that arrive in the HIM Department separately from the main record are often called **loose sheets**.

12. Required elements of a record that are missing are called **deficiencies**.

13. **Retention** procedures govern the storage of records, including duration, location, security, and access.

14. The data quality characteristic of data being present or existing in its entirety is **completeness**.

15. The process of recording elements into a collection device is called **data entry**.

16. The purpose of **concurrent analysis** is to review the chart while the patient is still being treated.

# Multiple Choice

1. Which of the following is a detective control?

   B. Reviewing a chart to ensure that medications were administered on a timely basis.

2. The coding system used to track diagnoses and procedures in an acute care setting is:

   A. ICD-9-CM

3. Which of the following is an example of a nomenclature?

   C. CPT-4

4. All of the following are steps in postdischarge processing EXCEPT:

   D. Concurrent Analysis

5. Which of the following is a preventive control?

   A. Alerting a physician that a patient is allergic to an ordered medication.

6. Upon review of a record, the analyst determines that the physician has not signed several progress notes. This record fails to reflect the data quality characteristic of:

   D. B&C

7. The JCAHO requires that acute care records be completed:

   C. Within 30 days of discharge

8. Acute care facilities are permitted to have delinquent records, but the number of delinquent records must not exceed:

   C. 50% of average monthly discharges

9. Which of the following is a corrective control?

   C. The HIM Department sends a physician a list of her incomplete charts.

10. Community Hospital, an acute care facility, is preparing for Joint Commission survey. The Chief Operating Officer is reviewing the following data from the Health Information Management Department:

    | Month | # Discharges | # Delinquent Records |
    |---|---|---|
    | January | 1000 | 450 |
    | February | 1200 | 600 |
    | March | 1100 | 500 |
    | April | 1100 | 600 |

    What is Community Hospital's average monthly discharges?

    C. 1100

11. How many delinquent records is Community permitted to have?

    C. 550

12. At the end of April, is Community Hospital in compliance with JCAHO rules?
    B. No

13. Control over records in process can be maintained using:
    C. Batch control record and central staging area

# 5

## Storage of Health Data

## *ANSWERS*

### Vocabulary

1. A digital form of the patient's paper health care record is called the **Computerized patient record**.

2. **Optical disk** is an alternative storage method for paper records using computer-based methods.

3. An **index** is used to identify or name a file or record so that it can be located in the computer-based health record.

4. The numerical file identification system used to identify an entire family's health record using one number and modifiers is called **family unit numbering**.

5. The length of time that a record must be retained is called the **record retention schedule**.

6. **Microfiche** and **microfilm** are alternative storage methods for paper records using plastic film.

7. A **Chart locator system** is used to identify the location of records within a facility.

8. The physical container used to store the paper-based health record is a **file folder**.

9. A **Computer-based patient record** is a compilation of patient health information, and various media forms all connected for fast access to patient information.

10. The **master patient index** contains patient and encounter information, often used to correlate the patient to the file identification.

11. A numerical patient record identification system, where the patient is given a new number for each visit, however with each new admission, the previous record is retrieved and filed in the folder with the most recent visit is called **serial-unit** numbering.

12. In a **Unit numbering** system the patient record is filed under the same number for all visits.

13. The filing method of organizing folders in numerical order is **straight numeric** filing.

14. A copier-like machine called a **scanner** is used to convert paper-based records into digital images for a computerized health care record.

15. A filing method in which the patient's MR# is separated into sets for filing, the first set of numbers are tertiary, the second set is called secondary, and the last set of numbers are called primary, is called **terminal digit** filing.

16. A numerical patient record identification system, which gives the patient a new number for each is called **Serial** numbering.

17. A physical file called an **outguide** is used to identify an alternate location of a file, in the paper-based health care record system.

## Multiple Choice

| | |
|---|---|
| 1. D | 5. D |
| 2. C | 6. B |
| 3. C | 7. A |
| 4. B | 8. D |

## Matching

| | |
|---|---|
| 1. I | 6. D |
| 2. J | 7. F |
| 3. C | 8. H |
| 4. B | 9. G |
| 5. E | 10. A |

# Uses of Health Data
## *ANSWERS*

## Vocabulary

1. **Brainstorming** is a quality improvement technique used to solicit participation and information from an entire group.

2. A supervisor and her team of employees are confronted with two solutions to a problem. Each solution involves time, money, and space; which quality management tool might the supervisor use to choose a solution: **decision matrix**.

3. A predetermined course of treatment for a patient with a particular diagnosis is known as a **clinical pathway**.

4. A method used to effectively manage patients during their hospitalization is known as **case management**.

5. Each month the Tumor Registry personnel are required to report the **incidence** of breast cancer for the facility. They report this statistic by determining the number of new cases of breast cancer for the month.

6. The method of reviewing patient information during hospitalization is known as **concurrent review**.

7. The **American College of Surgeons** preceded the JCAHO in the survey of hospitals against set standards.

8. Successful completion of a Medicare Conditions of Participation survey results in **certification** for the health care facility.

9. To improve quality according to a standard a health care facility may use **benchmarking**, the comparison of itself to that of a similar superior performer.

10. **Clinical pertinence** is the qualitative review of health care records to determine the appropriateness of care according to the patient's diagnosis.

11. Health information may be used in **litigation** to support the plaintiff's claim.

12. Thorough review of the patient's health information to determine pertinence, appropriateness, or compliance with standards is **qualitative analysis**.

13. **Mortality** refers to death within a population.

14. Health information may be analyzed to support a **marketing** campaign to promote the facility within its community.

15. Retrospective review of a product of a service is **quality assurance**.

16. The number of existing cancer cases reported by the tumor registry is known as **prevalence**.

17. A quality improvement effort regarding completion of the patient advance directive would require an **interdepartmental** team.

18. **Morbidity** refers to disease within a population.

19. A quality improvement effort regarding scanning of loose reports would require an **intradepartmental** team.

20. The alternative to quality assurance, **performance improvement** is an ongoing effort to improve processes within the health care facility.

21. The **risk management** process would be initiated following a patient fall from the bed, to gather information and coordinate the claim.

22. The monies collected by the health care facility from the payer is known as **reimbursement**.

23. Physicians may perform **research** to determine the cause or best treatment for a particular disease.

24. Ensuring appropriate, efficient, and effective patient care is a process of **utilization management**.

25. The review of the record performed postdischarge is known as **retrospective review**.

## Multiple Choice

1. D
2. A
3. C
4. B
5. C

6. B
7. D
8. A
9. A
10. C

## Matching

1. A
2. C
3. E

4. D
5. B

# 7

# Retrieval and Reporting of Health Information

## ANSWERS

## Vocabulary

1. The number of patients present in the health care facility, counted at the same time each day, is called the **census**.

2. All of the students registered for this class could be called a **population**.

3. Another name for a data illustration: **graph**.

4. The HIM department computer contains a **database**.

5. The subjective portion of a SOAP progress notes is **primary** data; also information obtained by a caregiver after observation of the patient.

6. Data processed into a meaningful format is known as **information**.

7. An **abstract** is a summary of the patient record.

8. UHDDS and UACDS are examples of a **data set**.

9. A report of a group of patients including their age is an example of **aggregate** data.

10. Diagnosis, physician, or procedure **indices** are used to organize and retrieve specific data from the HIM database.

11. The result of a query is also known as a **report**.

12. The Eye, Ear, Nose, and Throat hospital that performs ambulatory surgery must complete the **Uniform Ambulatory Care Data Set (UACDS)** on all of their patients.

13. Analysis, interpretation, and presentation of numbers is called **statistics**.

14. To study only the female students registered for this class, is to examine a **sample**.

15. Diamonte Hospital, an acute care facility, must complete the **Uniform Hospital Discharge Data Set (UHDDS)** on all patients discharged from the facility.

16. An organization of data elements in rows and columns is called a **table**.

17. When the clerk requests a report from a computer system, he/she is said to **query** the data base.

18. The diagnosis index is an example of **secondary** data.

19. A database of specific cancer or trauma information is an example of a **registry**.

## Multiple Choice

1. C
2. B
3. A
4. C
5. D

6. D
7. A
8. B
9. D
10. C

## Matching

1. A
2. H
3. G
4. D
5. E

6. J
7. C
8. B
9. I
10. F

# Confidentiality and Compliance
## *ANSWERS*

## Vocabulary

1. A permission that is given after the event to which the permission applies is **retrospective consent**.

2. Health information must not be disclosed inappropriately, because it is **confidential**.

3. Health records can be used as evidence in a court of law, because of the **business record rule**.

4. If a facility meets the standards set by a licensing or accrediting body, it is said to be in **compliance**.

5. In order for a court to hear a case, the court must have **jurisdiction** over the issue or the parties.

6. **Informed consent** is a permission given by a competent individual, of legal age, with full knowledge or understanding of the risks, potential benefits, and potential consequences of the permission,

7. Operational or procedural services that are provided by individuals or organizations who are not employees of the facility for which the services are being provided are said to have been **outsourced**.

8. Permission to perform a medical procedure or to release information generally requires the patient's **consent**.

9. Prospective consent for treatment is contained in the **Conditions of Admission**.

10. The ability to retrieve health information and provide it to requestors refers to **access**.

11. The **heresay rule** prohibits most testimony by parties not directly involved in the event.

12. The legal foundation for confidentiality is **physician-patient privilege**.

13. The party who initiates litigation is the **plaintiff**.

14. The **plaintiff** brings a lawsuit against the **defendant**.

15. The process of engaging in the legal proceedings of a lawsuit is **litigation**.

## Multiple Choice

1. All of the following are elements of the Business Record Rule EXCEPT:
   C. Records are kept in accordance with JCAHO standards

2. Conditions of Admission are an example of:
   A. Prospective consent

3. Federal court may have jurisdiction over all of the following EXCEPT:
   D. Amounts over $10,000

4. The practice of maintaining confidentiality in healthcare is based on:
   C. Physician-patient privilege

5. The new nursing supervisor is discussing with you her plans for the unit. She wants to hang a board on the wall of the nursing unit listing each patient's name, room number, working diagnosis, and medication schedule. You advise her that:
   B. This is a violation of confidentiality to display patient-specific information in a public place

6. An insurance company may obtain patient records by all of the following EXCEPT:
   B. Automatically, under 42CFR

7. A patient presents in the HIM Department requesting a copy of the record for his recent appendectomy. Upon inquiry, the patient reveals that, in addition to wanting a record of the operation, he had an allergic reaction to the anesthesia and wants to keep a record of this event in order to avoid a similar problem in the future. The patient should be advised to request a copy of:
   C. The Operative Report and the Anesthesia Records

8. Your facility charges a $10 search fee plus $1.00 per page to copy records up to 100 pages. All pages in excess of 100 are charged $.50 per page. Based on this schedule, what is the fee for a 125-page record?
   B. $122.50
      $10 search fee
      $100 for the first 100 pages (100 x 1.00)
      $12.50 for the last 25 pages (25 x .50)

9. The purpose of the JCAHO Steering Committee is to:
   D. All of the above

10. A valid consent for release of information contains all of the following EXCEPT:
    B. Patient's marital status

11. A 16-year-old patient presents in the emergency room for treatment of stomach pain. She is conscious, alert, and oriented. Of the following, who is the appropriate individual to sign the consent for treatment?
    A. The patient

## Matching

Number the steps in a civil lawsuit in their correct order:

5   1. Appeal

1   2. Complaint

2   3. Discovery

3   4. Pre-trial Conference

6   5. Satisfying the judgment

4   6. Trial

# 9

## Reimbursement
## *ANSWERS*

### Vocabulary

1. A data collection device that facilitates the accurate capture of ambulatory care diagnoses and services is an **encounter form**.

2. A health care provider applies to a payer for reimbursement by submitting a **claim**.

3. A savings account in which health care and certain child-care costs can be set aside and paid using pre-tax funds is a **flexible benefit account**.

4. Before a payer reimburses for a claim, there may be an amount for which the patient is personally responsible, called a **deductible**.

5. Fees or costs are also called **charges**.

6. HCFAs prospective payment system for hospital-based ambulatory care is based on **Ambulatory Patient Classifications**.

7. ICD-9-CM diagnosis and procedures codes are used to derive the DRG by following the flowchart in a **grouper**.

8. ICD-9-CM is coordinated and maintained by a group of four organizations collectively called the **Cooperating Parties**.

9. In Long-Term Care, the **Minimum Data Set** is used to determine the prospective payment.

10. In order to standardize and facilitate accurate billing, health care facilities maintain a database of all potential services to a patient called a **chargemaster**.

11. In return for the payment of a premium an **insurer (or insurance company)** assumes the risk of paying some or all of the cost of providing health care services to an individual or group of individuals.

12. Medicare uses **fiscal intermediaries** to process its claims and reimbursements.

13. Procedures and controls to ensure correct coding are part of a **coding compliance plan**.

14. Prospective payment for acute care is based on **Diagnosis-Related Groups**.

15. Reimbursement to a health care provider on a per-patient basis is **capitation**.

16. The amount paid to an insurance company by or on behalf of the insured is called a **premium**.

17. The process of determining the most accurate DRG payment is **optimization**.

18. The process of submitting claims or rendering invoices is called **billing**.

19. The systematic collection of specific charges for services rendered to a patient is called **charge capture**.

## Multiple Choice

1. The payer had an agreement with the physician to pay the 'usual and customary fee', less 10%. This is an example of:

   C. Discounted fee-for-service

USE THE FOLLOWING SCENARIO TO ANSWER QUESTIONS 2 AND 3:

The 82-year-old patient presented in the physician's office for a routine physical examination. He gave the receptionist two cards, evidencing his primary, government-funded insurance plan that pays for most of the bill and an additional, private plan that covers the remaining charges.

2. The patient's primary insurance is most likely:

   C. Medicare

3. The patient's secondary insurance is called:

   B. Wraparound plan

4. The physician charged the patient $75 for the office visit. The patient paid the physician $5 and the patient's insurance company paid the physician $70. This method of reimbursement is called:

   C. Fee-for-service

5. The physician charged the patient $75 for the office visit. The patient paid the physician $5 and the patient's insurance company paid the physician $70. The patient's portion of the payment is called:

   D. Co-payment

6. Title XVIII is the amendment to the Social Security Act that established:

   B. Medicaid

7. The payment rate established by an insurance company, based on its knowledge of the regional charges for a service are called:

   C. Usual and customary charges

8. Unlike prospective payment for acute care, long-term care prospective payment is on what basis?

   C. Per diem

9. An organization which insures as well as owns exerts employer control over the health care providers is a(n):

   A. Health Maintenance Organization

10. The department in a hospital that is primarily responsible for submitting bills or claims for reimbursement is:

    D. Patient accounts

# Matching

Match the definition on the left with the health insurance terminology on the right.

1. D

2. E

3. A

4. F

5. G

6. B or F

7. C

# 10

# Human Resource Management

## *ANSWERS*

## Vocabulary

1. An **FTE (full-time equivalent)** works 32-40 hours each week excluding over-time, earning full benefits as offered by the health care facility.

2. The **organization chart** is an illustration used to describe the relationship between departments, positions, and functions within an organization.

3. A formal list of the employee's responsibilities associated with their job is called a **job description**.

4. For the 2001-2002 fiscal year, the manager has set a **goal** to implement a document imaging system.

5. **Performance standards** are set guidelines explaining how much work an employee must complete.

6. In order to reach a desired goal the department must establish **objectives**, directions for achieving a goal.

7. As the new supervisor over the file area, release of Information and Assembly and Analysis, Sandra feels overwhelmed by the number of projects needing her attention. One way that Sandra may relieve the pressure form these projects is to **delegate** some of the projects to her employees.

8. A **job analysis** involves the review of a function to determine all of the tasks or components that make up an employee's job.

9. It is the responsibility of the employer to provide a safe work environment for the employee to perform his/her job function. One way that this can be accomplished is through design of an **ergonomic** work space.

10. The purpose of the organization documented in a formal statement is known as the **mission**.

11. The following is **Policy** of Diamonte Hospital, an equal opportunity employer. All new hires will be drug tested.

12. In the HIM department Judy, the Physician Record Clerk is responsible to Deenie the supervisor and Michelle the Director, this violates the **unity of command** principle.

13. **Productivity** is the amount of work produced by an employee in a given time frame.

14. A process that describes how to comply with a policy is a **procedure**.

15. Above and beyond the mission statement, a **Vision** sets a direction for the organization for the future.

16. Janet is a supervisor responsible for 8 coding employees, this statement represents Janet's **span of control**.

## Multiple Choice

1. C
2. D
3. B
4. C
5. C

6. C
7. D
8. A
9. C
10. B

## Matching

1. F
2. D
3. A
4. G

5. H
6. C
7. B
8. E

# 11

## Training and Development
# *ANSWERS*

## Vocabulary

1. **Credentials** indicate a person's specific professional qualifications.

2. The period of time, also known as a grace period, given to a new employee to learn the job and reach the performance standards associated with that job is known as the **probation period**.

3. **Minutes** are used to record the events, topics, and discussions of a meeting.

4. A name for the training provided to employees of an organization is **In-service**.

5. A general term for education, instruction, or demonstration of how to perform a job is known as **training**.

6. The term used to describe a training to familiarize a new employee to the job is **orientation**.

7. An **agenda** is used to organize the topics to be discussed during a meeting.

8. A written/typed communication tool used to communicate or provide information to members of an organization is a **Memorandum (Memo)**.

9. **Continuing education** may be required after attaining a position, credential, or degree intended to keep those persons knowledgeable in core content areas.

## Multiple Choice

1. B
2. C
3. D
4. A

5. B
6. C
7. B
8. A

## Matching

1. C
2. A
3. D

4. B
5. E